Anne Marie
Thank you for
all you do
to help others.
You have been
a true friend.
Love & Light
Carl

What People Are Saying About
Reducing Your Cancer Risk

I found the book so interesting that I could hardly wait to see what came next and I could not put it down until I had read it from cover to cover. So much of the information we may know or probably have heard about, however the way the author sets it out makes it new, tantalizing and exciting. I was thinking as I read through it, everyone can benefit from reading and using this information. He shares his interviews with many experts and it is so helpful how he lists their individual contact information. The book, I feel, covers all aspects of health, diet, exercise, meditation, prayer and much more coupled with a huge dose of 'Common Sense.' He puts it all in a way that is interesting to read and understand.

Rev Dr. Anne Marie Evers 'Best-Selling Author;' Ordained Minister; Doctor of Divinity; CEO of Affirmations International Publishing Company; Radio Host

---

The best of both worlds! Dr. Carl O. Helvie is the longest living lung cancer survivor having been given 6 months to live, 43 years ago. He has a Doctorate in Public Health, 2 Masters Degrees and is an RN Nurse Practitioner teaching nurses for years. With the combination of his personal experience and educational expertise he created the Carl O. Helvie Holistic Cancer Foundation. If there's a cancer survivor, author, educator, teacher, trainer from whom you want to learn, this is a must read from the only person representing the world of both cancer survivor and scientific education.

Kathy Sullivan, CNC

Using his public health and prevention education Dr Carl O. Helvie has spent his life teaching other how to prevent illnesses in his practice in homes and clinics, in books, blogs, on the radio and television, social media, and on his websites. His passion to help others led him to explore the work of Edgar Cayce almost fifty years ago that he integrated into an alternative holistic approach. This comprehensive book utilizes that approach and includes such topics as nutrition, exercise, herbs, antioxidants, anti-inflammatories, prayer, helping others, meditation, affirmations, gratitude, and many other concepts. You won't want to miss reading this book that could help you avoid a serious illness--cancer.

Jane Bohman. R.N., MPH

REDUCING YOUR CANCER RISK

(A Holistic Approach)

The Carl O Helvie Holistic Cancer Foundation

By Carl O. Helvie, R.N., Dr.P.H.

(A 44-Year Lung Cancer Survivor)

(Author of Best Seller - *You Can Beat Lung Cancer: Using Alternative/Integrative Interventions*)

ALL AUTHOR PROCEEDS FOR THE CANCER FOUNDATION

DISCLAIMER

This book details the author's experiences with and research findings published about preventing cancer. Although the author is a healthcare professional he is not your provider and does not know about your specific needs. .

The author and publisher are providing this book and its contents on an "as is" basis and make no representations or warranties of any kind with respect to this book or its contents. The author and publisher disclaim all such representations and warranties, including for example warranties of merchantability and healthcare for a particular purpose. In addition, the author and publisher do not represent or warrant that the information accessible via this book is accurate, complete or current.

The statements made about products and services may not have been evaluated by the U.S. Food and Drug Administration. They are not intended to diagnose, treat, cure, or prevent any condition or disease. Please consult with your own physician or healthcare specialist regarding the suggestions and recommendations made in this book.

Except as specifically stated in this book, neither the author or publisher, nor any authors, contributors, or other representatives will be liable for damages arising out of or in connection with the use of this book. This is a comprehensive limitation of liability that applies to all damages of any kind, including (without limitation) compensatory; direct, indirect or consequential damages; loss of data, income or profit; loss of or damage to property and claims of third parties.

You understand that this book is not intended as a substitute for consultation with a licensed healthcare practitioner, such as your physician. Before you begin any healthcare program, or change your lifestyle in any way, you will consult your physician or other licensed healthcare practitioner to ensure that you are in good health and that the examples contained in this book will not harm you.

This book provides content related to topics of physical, mental and spiritual health issues. As such, use of this book implies your acceptance of this disclaimer.

This book is dedicated to all individuals

interested in learning about

and making lifestyle

changes that might

save their life.

CONTENTS

Foreword

This book is down-to-earth, easy to understand and very informative. Dr. Helvie talks about implementing sensible, organic diet, exercise, vitamins and many other things for avoiding cancer. I just love his *'What to Do'* Sections which are filled with wonderful advice, ideas and suggestions. I found the whole book 'chuck full' of interesting findings and great advice that I can totally grasp and add into my life.

I found the book so interesting that I could hardly wait to see what came next and I could not put it down until I had read it from cover to cover. So much of the information we may know or probably have heard about, however the way the author sets it out makes it new, tantalizing and exciting. I was thinking as I read through it, everyone can benefit from reading and using this information. He shares his interviews with many experts and it is so helpful how he lists their individual contact information. The book, I feel, covers all aspects of health, diet, exercise, meditation, prayer and much more coupled with a huge dose of 'Common Sense.' He puts it all in a way that is interesting to read and understand.

If you are looking for help with anxiety, stress, depression and much more check out his 'What to Do'

Sections. He even shares websites where you can get a cook book, information on Nutrition and much more.

I give this book '5 Star' rating as it is the most comprehensive, complete, informative book ever on life, living and being the best you can be! Being a colon cancer survivor myself, I could relate to the information he so richly shares with the reader.

I also found the vitamin, supplement and other information most interesting and helpful. He talks about the importance of getting enough sleep (7-8 hours) to maintain the immune system and prevent cancer. He even suggests how to prepare yourself and your room for sleep with relaxation, meditation, prayer and as well infusing the room with Lavender or Jasmin Oil before sleeping.

I really like the way he suggests that folks quit smoking. He gives 12 helpful hints to help in the Quitting Process. I also love the affirmations he suggests, "I am happy to be a non-smoker. My lungs are clear and I breathe easily. I am now healthy and happy," all positive, uplifting statements designed to help the process. He adds the component of sound (music) to be used for soothing and healing during this period.

This is one-of-a-kind, a unique *Physical, Mental, and Spiritual Guide* with everything at your fingertips just waiting to be read and used.

He also states the importance of using positive affirmations and affirming in the now! I love the way Dr. Helvie tells about his prayer box and praying for others and how important creative visualization is to any positive process. He talks about the power of faith and gives suggestions on how to deal with negative situations in his 'What to Do' section. His books tells about healing, forgiveness and gratitude and again in his 'What to Do' section he provides hints, suggestions and examples sharing exactly how to do the processes.

You will also find an interesting section on meditation and again he shares suggestions, positive hints and statements on how to effectively visualize. He adds information about Optimism and Attitude Behavior and he covers the Fear of Flying situation which is very close to my heart and I use a very similar exercise when flying which works for me every time.

And it would not be complete without adding a section on Prayer and he shares 4 types of prayer – Petition/Thanksgiving/Praise and Confessional and describes each type of Prayer. Servicing others is a most important part to Dr. Helvie because he practices it daily and he excels at it. 'He walks his talk!' He also shares knowledge, information and suggestions on stress reduction which so many people struggle with daily and again his 'What to Do' Section gives wonderful, helpful easy suggestions.

I don't believe Dr. Helvie has overlooked anything! Once you read it, I know you will agree with me. I could go on and on – However my message is –

Please Buy the Book (Help the Cancer Foundation) and Yourself!

Affirmation Blessings

Rev Dr. Anne Marie Evers 'Best-Selling Author;' Ordained Minister; Doctor of Divinity; CEO of Affirmations International Publishing Company; Senior Radio Talk Show Host;

A Message from the Author

Please keep in mind that cancer, health, environment, and relationship information is an ever-changing process. As new research broadens our knowledge in these areas, changes in prevention and treatment follow. The author of this work checked with sources believed to be reliable in his effort to provide information that is complete, accurate, and reliable.

However, in view of the possibility of human error or changes in research finding, neither the author nor any publisher nor any other party who has been involved in the preparation or publication of the work is responsible for any error or omissions or for the results obtained from the use of such information. Readers are encouraged to confirm the information contained herein with other sources.

Considering ongoing new research and the resulting changes in cancer prevention and treatment knowledge this booklet will be updated periodically to reflect these changes. I hope you will find the information helpful in keeping cancer out of your lives.

Introduction

While writing a section on prevention for the Carl O Helvie Holistic Cancer Foundation website, I realized the importance of this content about things you can do to prevent cancer. As a cancer survivor and public health practitioner I knew from experience that it is less traumatic in one's life to improve diet, add exercise, prayer, meditation and other life style changes than it is to be disrupted by a diagnoses of cancer and, depending upon ones decision about treatment, be faced with pain and suffering for an extended period of time.

Thus, I decided to use the content developed for the website as a booklet also. A booklet has the advantage of having content all in one place instead of having to search for it on the website that is set up by categories such as research on physical aspects of cancer, research on mental/spiritual aspects of cancer, interviews with cancer doctors, interviews with cancer survivors and so forth. For each aspect of prevention such as EMF waves or nutrition I have reviewed research, explain how to use the information to prevent cancer, and often included a link to an interview with an expert.

I will be updating information in this booklet, and any additional ones, on the website, Current research and new interviews will also be added to the website as appropriate. In the process I will also share updates in newsletter with those who sign up for them on the website under the Contact button.

You will note that interventions for preventing cancer include gratitude, prayer, meditation, compassion and other mental/spiritual interventions not usually considered part of cancer treatment. As a pioneer in the use of a holistic cancer approach to cure cancer in 1974 my treatments included all natural physical interventions (no chemo, radiation or surgery) and also mental, and spiritual interventions. In addition, by using a holistic approach I never had a recurrence of cancer which is a common problem following many other treatments that omit the mental/spiritual dimensions of humans. Using this approach as a volunteer camp nurse for the Edgar Cayce organization from 1970 to 1974 and with other conditions than cancer and other individuals since then I know from experience that a holistic approach works so it is the basis of my radio show and the cancer foundation. Research over the past few years has confirmed the value of mental/spiritual interventions for cancer prevention/treatment and I look forward to the day when cancer is a thing of the past.

I wish to thank Dr. Joyce Adkins, my neighbor, and Kathy Sullivan, A *Facebook* friend and Advisory Committee member of the *Carl O Helvie Holistic Cancer Foundation*, who graciously reviewed and provided feedback and emotional support for this book.

REDUCING YOUR CANCER RISK: A HOLISTIC APPROACH

A. Brief Conceptual Framework for Cancer

Understanding cancer prevention activities begins with a framework of public health concepts to put the ideas into context. This framework provides an easier way to understand specific prevention-related strategies, research, and interviews with some of the national holistic leaders. A more complete framework can be found in Helvie's *Advanced Practice Nursing in the Community* that combines public health concepts with his Energy Theory of Nursing and Health and is available at Amazon's or Barnes & Noble.

Health/Illness/Cancer as Processes

Public health practitioners view health and illnesses (such as cancer) as processes that are dependent upon multiple factors in humans, the disease or disabling agent, and the environment that bring them (humans and the agent) together. Because of their interrelatedness it is possible for humans, communities, nations and the world to move up and down a health-illness continuum depending upon how well they deal with (resist or succumb) environmental/agent factors. If disease is to occur there must be a weakened host, a strong agent, and a favorable environment that brings them together. Thus, a three prong focus is used to move humans/communities/the world toward wellness on the health end of this continuum using interventions that:

1. Strengthen the person-increase the resistance of humans,
2. Weaken the risk factor-reduce the presence, forcefulness, or impact of the agent, and/or
3. Change the environment-make the environment less favorable/forceful for a human-agent interaction.

Intervening Points in the Process

It is possible to intervene with these multiple factors before or after humans interact with disease/ disabling agents in the environment. Intervening before humans interact with the environmental/ agent factors for cancer (before the illness) to make them more resistant and the environment/ disease agent less favorable is known as primary prevention. The major goal of primary prevention is to protect humans from cancer and help them maintain and improve their health and wellness. In other words, primary prevention aims to stop the disease from occurring through either changing individuals by making them stronger or by changing the environment to remove the risk factor or both.

Figure 1. Health/Illness Process Levels and Intervention Types

Health/Illness Level---------Healthy /// Early Disease /// Late Disease

Preventive Interventions---Primary--///Secondary------ ///Tertiary

---

Secondary prevention occurs further down a health-illness continuum when individuals have interacted with a disease agent in an unfavorable environment and experienced a negative effect or diagnoses of cancer. Secondary prevention is sometimes called early intervention. The goal here is to identify the disease as early as possible in order to reduce the length and severity of illness and produce a better outcome. Secondary prevention includes interventions for those with early cancer such as stage 1 or 2 cancer or before it has metastasized to other parts of the body where it would be more difficult to treat and the outcome would be less favorable. Secondary prevention can also include less invasive diagnostic tests such as the Navarro urine test and procedures such as breast and testicular self-examination.

Even further down the continuum is tertiary preventive interventions for those with the most severe illnesses. Tertiary prevention include treatment to contain the disease as well as to prevent the problem from returning after it has been treated. Also, in recent years, quaternary prevention has been introduced into health care which describes a process to prevent the results of unnecessary interventions or complications of excessive treatment. Our focus in this booklet is primary prevention and secondary and tertiary interventions will be presented at a later time.

Risk factors. Although there are no known agent factors in a holistic approach to cancer prevention such as bacteria and viruses found in acute communicable diseases there are risk factors that may trigger different types of cancer and that you should be aware of. For example, in a holistic approach (humans-agent-environment) lung cancer is more likely to occur in a person who is not exercising or keeping the immune system in balance, not eating a proper diet or getting adequate sleep and rest, who is missing prayer, meditation and relationship experiences and other lifestyle activities that help maintain wellness. In addition, cigarette smoke may be a high risk (trigger) because it is present in over 90% of all individuals with lung cancer and may makes a difference between having or avoiding lung cancer even when most other holistic factors (diet, exercise, supplements, prayer, meditation, and others) are positive. Likewise, there are variables in cigarette smokers that may account for the differences between those who have or do not have lung cancer. These may include an individual smoking many cigarettes containing heavy chemicals daily for many years vs one smoking a few, weak chemical cigarettes daily for a short period of time. Thus, the risk factor varies depending upon whether the agent or trigger is weak or strong as it interacts with other human and environmental factors to cause cancer. The same can be said for ultraviolet rays from the sun and/or tanning beds as they influences skin cancer. Frequent long time exposure for many years vs short term exposure of less intense rays (early morning or late afternoon) for a few years can impinge upon humans and produce cancer or not. Although the risks (agent/triggers) of different cancers will not be discussed here, be aware that these do exist and research those that are most important to you. I have included some triggers under individual or environmental factors below.

Every positive lifestyle activity helps. It may not be possible for you to make all of the positive changes identified below, but do what you can to reduce the risk of cancer. Each change can help tip the scale toward health and away from cancer. Some changes are more important than others as far as risk. For example, Dr Lise Alschuler in her interview (http://holisticcancerfoundation.com/) available under the Category Interviews with Doctors says 30 minutes a day of exercise can reduce cancer risk by 50% and proper diet can reduce it by 35%. Wow—these are big ones to focus on for change, if necessary. In addition, the triggers mentioned above are big ones. But do not ignore the other preventive interventions when you have time. Your efforts will be well rewarded.

Research findings. Research results for cancer causation/risk factors in the literature may seem to be contradictory. There are many reasons for these contradictions and a few will be identified here. First, research methodologies used in studies may vary and influence the findings. Some studies have large populations, use a random sample selection process to select subjects and controls, are prospective instead of retrospective or case studies, control for variables in subjects and controls and other factors that make the study results more reliable. When some or all of these and other research components are missing in a research study the results may vary, are usually less reliable, and cause variation with other reported results.

A second problem is that studies carried out on cells, or animals (usually precede clinical trials and human research) may have the findings falsely extrapolated to humans. This may happen as a result of research reviewed by individuals without a background in research in general or cancer specifically. If this information is repeated in other articles or posts on social media and is shared by others it may add to conflicting results in print if further studies on humans are different from those on cells, for example,---which does happen.

A third factor that causes conflicting results is the dishonesty of companies who sponsor research and have a vested interest. For example, those who sell soap, tooth paste and personal care products and make a profit from these items but also fund research on them may influence results that differ from findings if researchers are financed by different unbiased sources. Although there are many known instances, the following story of falsifying the results of the effects of laetrile at Sloan Kettering is well known and shows how this can be done.

Http://www.amazon.com/doctored-results-suppression-sloan-kettering-institute-ebook/dp/b00ib1pzqe

Therefore, you should review conflicting research results to your satisfaction before making decisions about using products. I tend to error on the side of avoiding them if there is any possibility that they are unsafe for me, my family, or friends.

Notify me. If you find glaring omissions in this overview of holistic cancer causing factors send me a note and I will research and add omissions and/or make changes as necessary on the website. I also plan to revisit this booklets periodically and add new content, interviews and research, and make corrections as necessary,

Apologies, if Necessary. The interviews with experts range from a few months to a few years old and because we are dynamic individuals some guests may have additional accomplishments to those listed. I have tried to include websites so you can review updates when necessary. If you need additional information on a guest interview or a website not listed, contact me and I will do my best to assist you.

B. Primary Prevention Interventions for Cancer

While there are three areas where primary prevention can be focused – the individual, the agent and the environment – the agent is most often interrelated with the environment. Because of the difficulty in considering an agent separately from the environment, it will be considered together as environmental factors in this book and we will focus on removing or limiting exposure to the environmental factor to weaken its risk. Following the discussion on environmental factors, there will be a discussion about ways to help individuals improve their resistance to potential exposure to agents or the environment. Many people find it easier to remove a risk from the environment than to make a change in lifestyle, but changing both the environmental exposure and the individual strengths is the most effective strategy.

Part 1. Environmental Factors (Reducing Environment/Agent Impact)

Preventive interventions in the areas of the environment and toxic agents include making environmental/agent factors less favorable for developing cancer. These strategies involve ways to avoid or prevent exposure to the risk factors as well as ways to mitigate or reduce the impact of the unavoidable factors. This section will discuss some of the toxic agents along with ways to reduce or mitigate your exposure or risk and the research behind the interventions.

✦1. A. EMF Waves

(These waves are most commonly found in computers, televisions, cell phones, microwaves, fluorescent lights, wired and wireless electronics, and even hair dryers.) Although research is contradictory some studies found cell phones can cause cancer of the brain and reproductive organs, and other sources of EMF waves may cause leukemia in children. In addition, the International Agency for Research on Cancer and the National Institute of Environmental Health Sciences EMF Working Group have classified EMF exposures as a possible human carcinogens

What to do:

√ Stay as far away from the source as possible.

√ Turn off electronics when not in use.

√ Do not use cell phone next to head, and do not store in pocket, or on body- connect them to an adapter when using.

√ Move WIFI out of bedroom or sleeping areas, if necessary and possible. If not, turn it off at night as it interferes with body rejuvenation and renewal that takes place during sleep.

Expert Interview for overall information on EMF waves and dangers listen to the interview with Dr David Carpenter below.

https://www.holisticcancerfoundation.com/intervie ws-others-treat-related-health-concerns-cancer/

Dr David O Carpenter is a public health physician and currently Director of the Institute for Health and the Environment at the University at Albany and also Professor of Environmental Health Science at the University of Albany in New York. He has carried out extensive research and has more than 370 peer-reviewed publications, 6 books and 50 reviews and book chapters to his credit. More can be found at:

http://www.albany.edu/sph/18918.php

₵1. B. Selected Toxic Chemicals

(These may be found in pesticides in agriculture, industry, homes, and gardens, industrial chemicals, waste, and waste byproducts, chemicals in consumer products that include building materials, furniture, food packaging, cosmetics; and pollution from coal fired plants, automobile exhaust and others).

Benzene. (This solvent is used in the chemical and pharmaceutical industries, and is released by oil refineries). Research shows it is linked to acute myeloid leukemia (AML) and chronic lymphocytic leukemia (CLL); breast cancer; lymphatic and hematopoietic cancers). For additional research data from the World Health Organization see the following:

http://www.who.int/ipcs/features/benzene

What to do:

√ When outside avoid, when possible, motor vehicle exhaust, industrial emissions, fumes at gas stations, and tobacco smoke.

√ When inside avoid inhaling glue, paint, furniture wax, and detergents.

√ Avoid hazardous waste sites.

√ Avoid drinking well water from sites near hazardous waste sites until inspected.

√ Wear protective equipment if working in industries using benzene.

√ Avoid tobacco smoke (see below).

♣Bisphenol A (BPA). This is a building block of polycarbonate plastic and is one of the most widely produced chemicals in the world. (It is used in hard plastics, food cans, drink cans, store receipts, and dental sealants.) Research shows it is an endocrine disrupter linked to breast and prostate cancers. For addition research (over 120 studies) go to the following link.

http://www.annualreviews.org/doi/abs/10.1146/annurev.publhealth.012809.103714?journalcode=publhealth

What to do:

√ Drink filtered water from a glass or stainless steel water bottles from companies like Nalgene or Sigg instead of bottled water in plastic that may leach from the container into water (especially during hot weather transporting)

√ Avoid eating microwavable meals in plastic containers. For example, try instead something like Amy's that uses a paper container. However, there are still questions about the use of plastic covers on Amy's foods...

√ Use stainless eating utensils, ceramic dishes and glass instead of plastic.

√Avoid foods packaged in metal cans or at least use only those marked BPA free lining or are packaged in paper cartons (soup).

√ Avoid using plastic storage containers for left over foods. Instead use glass containers with BPA free covers.

√ Instead of using a plastic coffee maker (or coffee maker with a plastic drip basket), switch to a French press, ceramic drip, or stainless steel electric percolator.

√ Consider exchanging plastic cling wrap for glass jars, or parchment paper to cover left over foods.

√ Keep plastic out of the freezer, microwave, or dishwasher because BPA leaches from plastics at a higher rate in hot or cold temperatures.

√ Avoid aluminum soda cans that may be lined with BPA.

√ Request "no receipt" when possible. The BPA may transfer to your fingers and leach into other paper products touched.

√ Ask your dentist about the sealants and compounds he uses in your teeth that may contain BPA.

⚜Tobacco and tobacco smoke. (This includes cigarettes, cigars, pipes, and smokeless tobacco such as snuff and chewing tobacco.) Research found tobacco products are a causal factor of cancer in lungs, mouth, larynx, nose, throat, esophagus, pancreas, stomach, cervix, kidney, bladder, ovaries, colorectal, and acute myeloid leukemia. It also increases the risk of lung cancer when combined with exposure to radon. Additional research data can be found at the following site:

http://www.cancer.org/cancer/cancercauses/tobaccoca ncer/tobacco-related-cancer-fact-sheet

What to do:

√ Stay away from all smoke-it can cause cancer in smokers and non-smokers around them.

√ If you use tobacco products, quit. Tobacco cessation techniques have been found to be helpful. Quitting can mitigate and sometimes reverse damage caused by smoking. It is never too late.

√ Smoking Cessation techniques are presented below.

Expert Interview – **Dr Scott McIntosh** is Director of the Greater Rochester Tobacco Research Program and Associate Director of the Smoking Research Program and Associate Professor, Division of Social and Behavioral Medicine, Community and Preventive Medicine at the University of Rochester in New York. His research is on self-help interventions for smoking cessation and behavioral change with various populations and he has received numerous research grants and published many articles and book chapters. Last year he received the American Cancer Society's first "Fight Back" award for his commitment for helping people quit smoking and reduce the cancer incidence. One of his web sites is linked next followed by our interview.

http://www.myclearhorizons.com Interview link below.

https://www.holisticcancerfoundation.com/intervie ws-others-treat-related-health-concerns-cancer/

↳Formaldehyde. (It has been found in building and home decoration products, auto exhausts, preservatives, and disinfectants). Research has linked it to leukemia and nasopharyngeal cancer. More information on cancer and formaldehyde from the National Cancer Institute can be found at:

http://www.cancer.gov/about-cancer/causes-prevention/risk/substances/formaldehyde/formaldehyd e-fact-sheet

What to do:

√ Avoid auto exhausts.

√ Avoid cigarette smoke indoors.

√ Buy formaldehyde free furnishings and construction materials when building and furnishing houses.

Methyl Bromide. (It is used to sterilize soil before planting strawberries <u>and</u> tomatoes, including organic ones, and for fumigation of ham and pork products. It was phased out as a pesticide in most countries in early 2000's but continued in the USA until at least 2017 when it is to be phased out worldwide). It is considered a potential occupational carcinogen by OSHA and can cause cancer and death depending upon the concentration. It has been related to prostate cancer risk.

<u>What to do:</u>

√ Avoid or limit strawberries and other foods known to be contaminated.

√ Research to determine if it is discontinued in 2017 before reintroducing these foods into your diet. Ask your local farmers if they use this chemical before planting strawberries and tomatoes. If not, use the foods because they are very healthy.

Polybrominated diphenylethers (PBDS). (This can be found in flame retardants in furniture, computers, electronics, medical equipment, and mattresses). It is an endocrine disrupter that may cause liver cancer.

<u>What to do:</u>

√ Avoid furniture and mattresses with flame retardants.

√ Check out computers and other electronics before buying.

Multiple chemicals. Please see the discussion on multiple metals/chemical overload below.

✓Triclosan. (This can be found in Colgate's total toothpaste and some antibacterial soap, cosmetics and other personal products.) Although research is contradictory animal studies show it may cause endocrine- disruption, may act in a way similar to bisphenol (BPA) discussed previously, and may promote liver and other cancers. Additional research at:

http://www.niehs.nih.gov/news/newsletter/2015/1/scie nce-triclosan/ Pressure has been put on the EPA to ban the product: http://www.psr.org/environment

What to do:

√ The FDA banned Triclosan and 17 other chemicals in personal care products in September, 2016 but companies have 1 year to comply.

√ Research your personal care products and avoid those with Triclosan as an ingredient, if desired.

√ Although ingredients in products change over time as a result of public scrutiny and the lists of contaminated products are long the following guidelines are a start.

√ Research especially soap products that are liquid in dispensable containers that often have Triclosan. .

√ Look closely at germ free products that say germ killing or antibacterial.

√ Go organic when possible. A good choice for soap is Vi-Tae antibacterial soap (certified organic) that is advertised as natural and aromatherapy herbal bars. Few toothpaste products are organic. *Toms of Maine* (a popular product) is marked natural (not organic) and some of their products contains fluoride (see toxic metals below). Others are fluoride free. None contain Triclosan. However, some also contain carrageenan (see discussion below under additives). So again review ingredients. Dr Bronner's all-one tooth paste seems like a better choice because it is 70% organic, does not contain Triclosan, fluoride, or carrageenan. Himalayan Neern and Pomegranate toothpaste is also a good choice-an organic herbal product with no fluoride, or Triclosan but it does contain carrageenan.

√ Avoid also Triclocarban ingredients in products because of similar actions,

Expert Interview on chemicals and cancer. Listen to the interview with Dr Harry Milman below.

Dr Harry Milman is a PhD consulting toxicologist and expert witness and president of ToxNetwork.com. He has assisted as an expert in over 250 civil and criminal cases involving drug overdoses, pharmacy errors, exposure to toxic chemicals and carcinogens, and assaults. He is often quoted in newspaper and magazine articles and has appeared as a toxicology expert on television news broadcasts. Prior to becoming an expert witness, Dr. Milman was a scientist at the US National Cancer Institute, NIH, and a senior toxicologist at the US Environmental Protection Agency. He has published five scientific books including the widely acclaimed *Handbook of Carcinogen Testing* and over seventy research papers. *A Death at Camp David* is his first novel. He lives in the Maryland suburbs of Washington, DC More information is available at the next link followed by our interview.

http://www.toxnetwork.com/

**https://www.holisticcancerfoundation.com/intervie
ws-others-treat-related-health-concerns-cancer/**

41. C. Selected Toxic Metals

(These may be found in tooth paste, tooth fillings,
antiperspirant, home pipes and walls, occupational
settings, food and water, and other environmental
sources.) A new service in June, 2016 for testing
heavy metals, minerals, and elements such as
aluminum, magnesium, iron, potassium, copper and
others in food, protein powder, personal care products,
water and other items is available at:

http://cwclabs.com/

Aluminum. (It may be found in antiperspirants).
Research data on risk of aluminum for breast cancer is
mixed. Additional data at:

http://www.prevention.com/beauty/skin-care/does-
aluminum-antiperspirants-cause-cancer-and-
alzheimers

What to do:

√ Avoid antiperspirants with aluminum.

√ Use aluminum free antiperspirants/
deodorants-Toms of Maine have some but read

the label because not all Tom's products are aluminum free.

⚜*Asbestos.* (This may be found in walls, ceiling, and floors of older houses.) Research shows asbestos can cause mesothelioma and lung cancer as well as cancer of the bronchus, trachea, digestive organs, and peritoneum. See the following research data from the National Cancer Institute:

http://www.cancer.gov/about-cancer/causes-prevention/risk/substances/asbestos/asbestos-fact-sheet

What to do:

√ Have your house assessed for the presence of asbestos. It may be o.k. if it is present but not moved or exposed to humans.

√ If removal is needed, hire a profession to do the job.

⚜*Fluoride.* (It is found in the water supply of many communities and in dental products such as tooth paste and mouth wash.) Most research finds it dangerous and the FDA now requires a poison warning on all fluoride toothpastes sold in the U.S. In addition, tens of millions of people throughout China and India suffer serious crippling bone diseases from drinking water with elevated levels of fluoride. There are inconsistent research findings regarding a risk of fluoride for a rare type of bone cancers known as osteosarcoma especially in teen age boys, as well as bladder and lung cancer. For additional research on fluoride and cancer see:

http://fluoridealert.org/issues/health/cancer/

<u>What to do</u>:

√ Decide for yourself based upon your collected data whether you choose to do the following that I highly recommend:

√ Drink filtered water that removes fluoride and use non-fluoride tooth paste and mouth washes. Toms of Maine has some fluoride free tooth paste and a better choice if you can find it is Earthpaste, an all-natural toothpaste.

Lead. (In the past lead in interior paint chipped and children ate the paint chips. This may still be common in older homes that may also have lead water pipes. It is also found in water and soil, lipstick, and occupational sources). There is a weak connection to cancer but if it occurs, it may be found in lungs, stomach, gliomas and other sites. See additional research studies at:

https://www.ncbi.nlm.nih.gov/pmc/articles/PMC41442 70/

<u>What to do</u>:

√ If lead is found in old paint in homes, remove it if children are present.

√ Remove lead pipes and blinds in homes.

√ Wear protective clothing and limit exposure time if there is occupational exposure.

√ Avoid products such as lip stick that may contain lead.

Mercury. (Mercury can be found in the mercury-amalgam fillings in your teeth, lip stick, flu vaccines, power plant contaminants, batteries, fish/seafood, skin care products, florescent light bulbs, old fashion thermometers and more.) Research studies found that mercury in high levels depletes the immune system and is a factor in kidney, lung and brain diseases. There is not enough research evidence to determine mercury causes cancer or that mercury in fish or dental fillings are unsafe for most people according to the America Dental Assn. and most research studies. However, one study by the Communicable Disease Center found that individuals with more amalgam fillings had significantly higher levels of chronic health conditions such as multiple sclerosis, epilepsy, migraines, mental disorders, diseases of the nervous system, diseases of the thyroid, cancer, and infectious diseases than those with less or none. Also, read the convincing evidence in the following link. As a public health practitioner/educator I recommend doing what you can to avoid cancer or any other disease.

https://www.cancertutor.com/advdental/

<u>What to do</u>:

√ Have amalgam-mercury fillings removed by a specialist, if needed. See interviews with Bill Henderson and with Dr Vladimir Gashinsky below.

√ Avoid skin care products containing mercury.

√ If you live around a coal powered power plant be alert to symptoms of mercury poisoning and take action, if needed. If you work in a plant use protective clothing and equipment.

√ Use published hazard cautions for removing and disposing of a broken thermometer or florescent bulb to eliminate pollution in the environment.

√ Avoid flu injections and vaccines or extend the period between them if given in a series, if possible. Find alternative non-metal ways to protect yourself from the flu and other illnesses. Use a holistic approach to build up the immune system by following a protocol of a proper diet, exercise, having daily prayer, avoiding crowds in winter, and using natural products such as colloidal silver, oregano oil, elderberry syrup, and extra whole food vitamin C for viral, bacterial, and other infections.

√ Avoid eating large fish (large fish eat smaller fish and thus have higher levels of mercury) and limit all fish/seafood. Look for recommended weekly allowances based upon your age/ condition. .

√ Although research is contradictory I recommend avoiding farm grown fish because of potential cancer producing toxins, inflammatory and chemical contaminants.

Expert Interview on mercury and teeth. Listen to the interview with Bill Henderson and Dr Vladimir Gashinsky below.

Bill Henderson was a best-selling author of three books on the natural healing of cancer and coached over 3500 cancer patients. More information can be found at the next link followed by my interview with Bill.

http://www.beating-cancer-gently.com/

https://www.holisticcancerfoundation.com/intervie ws-others-treat-related-health-concerns-cancer/

Dr Vladimir Gashinsky has been in private practice at his Millburn, NJ office for over a decade, and earned his doctorate degree from NYU College of Dentistry, after which he became their clinical faculty leader. He is also proud to be an Accredited Member of the International Academy of Oral Medicine and Toxicology (IAOMT) and Certified in Ozone Dentistry through the ACIMD and is now pursuing his ND degree. He has extensive training in homeopathy and nutrition. Dr. Gashinsky spends countless hours doing continuing education with like-minded practitioners to keep up with new medical and technical developments in his field which he is bringing to his practice to help his patients achieve the best holistic dental care possible. Dr. Gashinsky has the distinction of having won the Eugene Rothschild Memorial Award from the New York Academy of Oral Rehabilitation. More information available below followed by his interview.

www.holisticdentalcenternj.com

https://www.holisticcancerfoundation.com/intervie ws-others-treat-related-health-concerns-cancer/

Radon. (It may be found in countertops, and in house seepage from external sources.) Research found radon to be a factor in some lung cancers. More research on radon and cancer at the National Cancer Institute site follows.

http://www.cancer.gov/about-cancer/causes-prevention/risk/substances/radon/radon-fact-sheet

What to do:

√ Have your house evaluated for the presence of radon when buying or selling. See testing for presence of radon below.

√ If you are buying a new home, ask if radon resistant materials were used in construction. See radon resistance below.

√ Have your home repaired if the radon level is four picocuries or higher.

√ Radon levels less than that pose a threat but can usually be reduced by one of the following procedures.

√ Air pressure differences between inside and outside air drives the radon into the house through cracks. Thus, 1) Seal floors to eliminate its entry. 2) Reduce radon levels before it enters the house by: using an under house sump system that collects radon in an area the size of a bucket and vents it outside; improve ventilation under suspended timber floors; and install positive ventilation systems that increase pressure and prevent seepage into the house. 3. Remove radon if it enters the house.

√ Testing for the presence of radon can be done by the homeowner or a specified radon tester, often a home inspector. Two types of radon test are available: active or passive. <u>Passive</u> devices are put in a home for a specified period of time and then sent to the lab for analysis. They are usually inexpensive and can be purchased at: <u>www.testproduct.com/safecart</u>. <u>Active</u> devices require power to function unlike passive devices and provide continuous monitoring, measuring, and recording of the amount of radon in the home. Both short term and long term methods are available. Short term testing uses a device in the home for two to ninety days whereas long term testing continues for more than ninety days.

√ Radon resistant materials can be used when a home is built and prevents radon seepage. You may wish to discuss this with your builder if you live in a high radon area of the country. A gas permeable layer is placed beneath the flooring or slab that allows radon to move freely under the house. This consists of four inches of clean gravel and is used only in homes with basements or slabs but not with a crawl space. Next, place clear plastic sheeting over the permeable layer and under the slab to help prevent seepage from the radon. Next, seal and caulk all below grade openings in the foundation and walls. Next, run a three or four inch PVP vent pipe from the gas permeable layer through the house to the roof to safely vent the radon and other gases to the outside. Place an electrical junction box in the attic so that a vent fan can be wired and installed.

Multiple metals/chemical overload. Research is very limited and controversial but most studies report the healthy body will adequately detox usual chemicals and metals on its own but detoxing may be necessary for alcoholics, or for removing lead from children. Many non-health professionals and some health professionals believe our bodies become overloaded with toxic metals and chemicals from our air, water and food and the body is thus unable to dispose of them properly. When this happens they may develop cancer. They believe that periodic detoxing will help prevent this process. You may wish to use one or more of the following mild interventions identified in the what to do list. The following is a typical overview of detoxing and research written by traditional medicine that is opposed to detoxing.

https://www.sciencebasedmedicine.org/the-detox-scam-how-to-spot-it-and-how-to-avoid-it/

NB: this was written_by an author with a masters of business administration and a doctorate in pharmacology. He is a pharmacist (who wants to sell drugs-right!)

What to do:

√ First, get rid of some of the toxins in your diet/home including GMO foods, pesticide laden foods, processed foods, and toxic products (see the section on chemicals and metals). Go organic and whole food (see section on nutrition.)

√ Exercise enough to sweat or sit in a sauna for 20 minutes. Try to sweat at least 20 minutes each day.

√ When I had lung cancer in 1974 my doctor recommended a detox of only juices one day a month as part of my natural treatment protocol. Try it and see how you feel. Of course, a vegan diet with high amounts of raw fruit and vegetables helped the process.

√ Include detoxing foods in your diet such as fruits and vegetables. Have a lemon drink when you arise in the morning. Use juicing during the day to include greens and an array of colorful vegetables-also include turmeric, garlic, and oregano in your diet but see precautions first if you have health issues.

√ Deep breath during the day to stimulate the lymphatic system and increase the absorption of fruits and vegetables.

√ Stay well hydrated to remove toxins.

√ Edgar Cayce recommended a 3 day apple diet for detoxing. He specified only apples, water and plenty of rest. The apples were to be of the Jenneting variety (Jonathan or Delicious work great). Eat at least 5 or 6 a day. At the end of the 3 days take 2 or 3 teaspoons of cold pressed olive oil. He said that if you are on an oil restricted diet you could extend the diet of apples to 4 or 5 days.

√ It is believed that toxic metals will replace needed minerals when they are in short supply. It is possible to test eight essential minerals and increase them regularly as needed. The Body Bio liquid mineral test kit, instructions and minerals are available at:

http://livesuperfoods.com/liquid-mineral-taste-test-kit-bodybio.html

√ For more specific detoxing of organs, google Dr Judy Seeger and attend one of her webinars. You may also listen to her interview/webinars below.

<u>Expert Interview</u>: Naturopathic doctor, **Dr Judy Seeger** has more than thirty years in the field of alternative medicine and was the director at River of Life Health Center, a Holistic Health Clinic. As director she developed a *Two Step Health Plan* System that increases health and quality of life for patients with skin, lung, breast, ovarian, prostate, liver, colon, brain and pancreatic cancers. Dr. Seeger specializes in and offered nearly every clinically proven natural healing therapy like Hyperbaric Oxygen Therapy, Ozone Therapy, Colon Hydrotherapy, Herbal Therapy, and Enzyme Therapy. She's also authored two books, both of which are available exclusively in an electronic format. These books, *The Ultimate Guide to Natural Cancer Cures* and *Shatter Your Gallstones* are insightful extensions of Dr. Seeger's brilliant and talented knowledge base. Along with these books, she's also created training videos, instructional CD's, conducted teleseminars and webinars. Most recently Dr. Seeger is conducting groundbreaking herbal research in the Amazon Rainforest. She's also continually developing mass media outreach programs. Her Cancer Winner Radio show is a broadcast radio show during which she interviews former cancer patients who overcame their disease using alternative therapies. She's also hosting an online television show, Cancer Answers. In these online video segments experts in the field of cancer research will share experience and advice with patients. Currently she is

developing webinars on detoxing for patients following chemo or radiation. More information is available below followed by her interview on detoxing.

http://beatcancer.org/medical-advisory-board/dr-judy-seeger

https://www.holisticcancerfoundation.com/intervie ws-cancer-doctors/

NB: Many people consider vaccines to be dangerous because they contain toxic substances that are potentially carcinogenic. This may be especially true from the interactions with one another when given close together without research on the effect of these interactions. For example, children today receive over 65 doses of 16 different vaccines before age 18. No research has been carried out on the interaction of the toxic substances in multiple vaccines and its influence on health. In addition, vaccines may contain formaldehyde and mercury (known carcinogen) as well as aluminum (possible carcinogen) and other toxic substances.

An interesting concept is presented by Ed Kane in the following videos. He believes that when we are low on specific minerals the heavy metals may take over and cause harm to the body. He has developed a taste test kit of 8 essential minerals to help individuals maintain a proper level of these minerals. I recommend this easy and inexpensive way to maintain proper levels of the essential minerals. The videos follows:

http://www.bodybio.com/content.aspx?page=BodyBio WellnessVideoLibrary

http://www.bodybio.com/content.aspx?page=TraceMi nerals-PartTwo

http://www.bodybio.com/content.aspx?page=TraceMi nerals-PartThree

The Test Kit is available for purchase at Amazon:

https://www.amazon.com/BodyBio-MTK-Liquid-Mineral-Test/dp/B0058A9T4K/ref=sr_1_1_a_it?ie=UTF8&qid =1491835121&sr=8-1&keywords=mineral+test+kit+by+bodybio

♦1. D. Ultraviolet Rays (UV)

(Overexposure of ultraviolet rays from the sun and tanning beds.) Research finds a link to skin cancer including melanoma from over exposure of sunshine and tanning beds. Additional research information at:

http://www.cancer.org/cancer/cancercauses/radiatione xposureandcancer/uvradiation/uv-radiation-does-uv-cause-cancer

What to do:

√ Avoid midday sunshine, if possible.

√ Limit your time in the sun but get sunshine often enough to meet vitamin D requirements. (Research shows that low levels of vitamin D are a risk factor for melanoma and other types of cancer).

√ If long term sun exposure is necessary wear protective clothing.

√ Eat lots of antioxidant foods that will decrease damage by the sun.

√ Sunscreen use is controversial because of the chemicals in the sunscreens and its efficacy in preventing sun rays. Most research seems to advocate sun screen but do your own research. The following important information will help you pick a safer sunscreen,

http://articles.mercola.com/sites/articles/archive/2014/06/04/ewg-sunscreen-guide.aspx

√ Consider an oral sun screen for protection against cancer. The latest research (2016) shows nicotinamide boosts energy levels in cells that allows them to repair DNA following ultraviolet radiation damage and reduces the risk of skin cancer by 23%. It is best used in combination with red orange extract and polypodium leucotomos extract to reduce inflammation. For extended exposure also use a topical sun screen.

√ Dr Mercola recommends an oral sunscreen called Ataxanthin, a carotenoid that will protects the skin from the sun. It is one of the most powerful antioxidants and he recommends starting with 2 mg daily.

Part 2. Individual Factors-Physical Aspects (Lifestyle Choices to Increase Your Resistance)

Besides environmental changes identified above there are things you can do to reduce the risk of cancer by making your body/mind/spirit more resistant to cancer. Some of these activities are identified below under two categories: physical aspects (below) and later under Part 3 are mental/spiritual aspects.

2. A. Physical Activity

(These may prevent obesity, reduce inflammation and hormone levels, improve insulin resistance and immune system functioning). Research has found a relationship between exercise and reduced risk of colon cancer (40-50%), breast cancer (30-40%), uterine cancer (38-46%) and lung cancer. Additional research information at:

http://www.cancer.gov/about-cancer/causes-prevention/risk/obesity/physical-activity-fact-sheet

What to Do:

√ Exercise 30 minutes daily for 5 or 6 days a week. The more vigorous and longer the exercise the lower the risk of cancer but research has not shown whether or not there is a limit.

√ Exercises may include walking, swimming, biking, running and others including gym exercises.

₵2. B. Fluids: Water and Milk

(Fluids including water and milk come in different containers and have different processes carried out before you receive them). Research shows some chemicals found in drinking water from the tap or bottle water can be cancer producing. Some chemicals in bottled water may include BPA, phthalates, and arsenic causing endocrine disruption and breast and prostate cancers, as well as bladder, kidney, liver, nasal and others, and tap water with fluoride, prescription drugs and other pollutants cause multiple diseases. Milk may contain genetically modified growth hormones, blood, pus, antibiotics, pharmaceuticals, and other pollutants. Drinking milk has been linked to breast, prostate, ovarian, and colon cancers).

<u>*Water*</u>: What to do:

√ Avoid drinking tap water w/chemicals (See the discussion on fluoride in water under environmental factors---chemicals above)

√ Drink filtered water from a glass or from stainless steel water bottles from companies like Nalgene or Sigg instead of bottled water in plastic bottles that may leach bisphenol (BPA) from the container into water (See the discussion on environmental factors -chemicals above)

√ Install a filtration system for drinking water.

√ Install filtered shower heads on your showers.

√ Drink at least 8 glasses of water daily to nourish the cells and remove toxins.

√ Although controversial some people advocate maintaining an alkaline balance in the body to reduce the risk of cancer. Because this belief is so widespread some time will be devoted to it. The American Institute for Cancer Research (http://preventcancer.aicr.org/site/news2?id=134 41) says "the unsubstantiated theory of alkalinity and cancer is based on lab studies that suggest cancer cells thrive in an acidic (low pH) environment, but cannot survive in alkaline (high pH) surroundings. While these findings are accurate, the research applies only to cells in an isolated lab setting. Altering the cell environment of the human body to create a less-acidic, less-cancer-friendly environment is virtually impossible." They continue on to say different parts of the body maintain different acid-alkaline levels and it would be dangerous to some organs in the body to force change even if it were possible. The process of maintaining body levels within a range and how change in a part affects other parts of the body and the whole that eventually can lead to dysfunction of parts and the whole body is well described in Helvie's energy theory books.

Http://www.curetoday.com/publications/cure/20
15/summer-2015/acid-
test?p=2#sthash.os4wp8oq.dpuf

In the link above The Canadian Cancer Society says the body has a complex system that makes sure the blood stays in its healthy, slightly alkaline range. If the blood becomes too acidic or too alkaline, the body automatically corrects this on its own. Your blood may become slightly more acidic or alkaline after eating certain foods but it will stay within the healthy range without a special diet. Dr Mitchell L Gaynor, a medical oncologist says "all of these 'high alkaline' foods are good, not because you're changing the pH of your blood, but because they're promoting good bacteria in your gut. Dr Andrew Weil and most scientists agree.

√ If you choose to alkalize parts of the body such as the gut it might be done using simple food sources or more expensive equipment. 1) Many people squeeze 3 fresh organic lemons and add water and a bit of Stevia, if preferred, and drink it first thing in the morning. It is very good for alkalizing the GI system.

Some people use a product called X2O made by Xooma. You add packets of this product made from magnesium, calcium and other trace minerals to your drinking water for the day, shake and let sit for 20 minutes before drinking throughout the day. It helps maintain alkalinity. Directions for mixing are on the bottle and the product is available locally or at the following.

http://www.xooma.com/products-product-x2o.php

Another product advocated by Bill Henderson is the alkaline water filters that vary in price from under $100 to around $3000. The more expensive models allows you to set your desired pH level. Information is available at:

http://www.ancient5.com

Note: some believe that candida, a potentially serious GI tract condition that can lead to leaky gut and IBS, is a result of an alkaline gut environment. Thus, maintaining an alkaline gut to prevent cancer may be causal of another serious health challenge-the fungal form of candida, and there is also a concept of fungus as causal of cancer. So do your research. As discussed above, if you change one part of the body it will affect other parts and the whole and when the body is no longer able to adapt, illness may result.

Note 2: Worry, anger and other negative emotions will also increase acidity temporarily in some body fluids;

Note 3: Vegans and vegetarians who omit meat and other acid forming foods may have a slightly lower pH in the gut (blood) temporarily following meals than those eating the standard American diet (SAD),

My personal preference: I believe in the old adage of KISS—keep it simple stupid. Thus, use a lemon drink in the morning or other foods, and overcome negative emotions but avoid the machines that claim to change your pH body level drastically. Although changing the body pH level physiologically is not possible according to researchers it may change the gut/blood pH temporarily and cause the body to work harder to revert to the normal pH level. I believe this stress on a body part can eventually lead to an imbalance in the whole body. And once you have an imbalance or disease some of the more harsh methods may be required to revert to a normal pH of some body parts.

Milk - What to do:

√ Replace cow's milk with a substitute such as rice milk, almond milk, hemp milk or raw goat's milk (check for added chemicals that may be carcinogenic as discussed above). .

√ If you choose to continue drinking cow's milk make sure it is non-genetic modified organic raw milk.

√Reduce cheese intake and eat organic goat's milk cheese.

∉2. C. Nutrition

(The standard American diet (SAD) is rich in animal proteins and fats, high in cholesterol and saturated fats, high in processed foods and sugar, and low in fiber, complex carbohydrates, and vegetables, and often contains genetically modified organisms, pesticides, growth hormones and other contaminants). Research shows that the standard American diet (SAD) can be a causal factor in cancer and an improved diet is a major factor in overcoming/preventing cancer.

What to do:

√ Eat plenty of fresh organically grown fruits and vegetables especially raw ones in salads and juicing. .

√ Eat smaller amounts of grains and nuts.

√ Use a good source of fat such as extra virgin cold pressed organic olive oil for low/no temperature food preparation and extra virgin cold press coconut oil or other high heat oils for high temperature cooking. If you use canola oil or sunflower oil make sure they are organic. 90% of all canola oil is genetically modified. Check labels because potato chips, popcorn, and other prepared foods may be prepared with canola oil.

√ Eat organically grown foods as much as possible and locally grown if you know the farming practices of your source. If you can't afford organic fruits and vegetables avoid the dirty dozen, a list developed each year of those with the most pesticides and chemicals. In 2015 this list included apples, peaches, nectarines, strawberries, grapes, celery, spinach, sweet bell peppers, cucumbers, cherry tomatoes, imported snap peas and potatoes. On the other hand eat those that are the clean fifteen: avocado, cantaloupe, onions, mangos, eggplant, frozen sweet peas, cabbage, kiwi fruit, pineapple, sweet potatoes, papaya, sweet corn, cauliflower, asparagus, and grapefruit. (Note that some of these are mainly GMO foods such as corn and papaya so again check for organic.) For updates of the dirty dozen and clean fifteen go to:

https://www.ewg.org/foodnews/?gclid=CKOf_
Y2S0c8CFc6Xfgod8hMC5Q

√ Eat anti-inflammatory foods to curb body inflammation such as fatty fish (mackerel, salmon, tuna, and sardines), whole (not refined) grains, dark leafy vegetables (spinach, kale, broccoli, collard greens), nuts (especially almonds and walnuts), and soy (controversial-in the form of tofu, soy milk, and edamame). Dr Andrew Weil has an anti-inflammatory diet that can be viewed at:

http://www.drweil.com/drw/u/art02012/anti-
inflammatory-diet

Also see the expert interview on nutrition and anti-inflammation with Julie Daniluk below.

√ Eat foods that are high in anti-oxidants such as berries (blackberries, strawberries, blue berries, raspberries), beans (pinto and red), Russet potatoes, red delicious apples, walnuts, cloves, spinach, cherries, grapes, prunes, and cranberries. (See information about strawberries above under chemicals→ methyl bromide). Also see expert interview on antioxidants and cancer with Dr Kedar N Prasad below.

√ Avoid farm grown products including salmon because of harmful toxins. .

√ Research the safety of additives in foods. For example, carrageenan used as a thickening in almond milk, baby formulas, some foods and personal care products is controversial in terms of safety. Animal research is divided on its safety and although you will find it in baby formula in the USA, it is not allowed in Europe.

√ Avoid eating large fish that eat smaller fish and, thus, have concentrate mercury levels. Limit number of servings weekly. If pregnant research further for guidelines.

√ Avoid genetically modified foods, Always look for the GMO free triangle on the box. If you cannot afford all GMO foods avoid the following that are most often GMO grown--- soy, cotton, canola, corn, sugar beets, Hawaiian papaya, alfalfa, and squash—both zucchini and yellow. In addition, many of these foods appear as added ingredients in a large amount of the foods we eat. For example potato chips and popped corn are often fried in canola oil and 90% of all canola oil is genetically modified. If you like canola oil Trader Joes has an organic canola oil. If you want occasional potato chips fried in coconut oil (non-GMO) try Jackson purple potato chips fried in coconut oil.

Http://jacksons-honest.myshopify.com/products/purple-heirloom-potato-chips?variant=7380785347

See the GMO expert interview below.

√ Eat simple sugars such as pies, cakes, candy, and ice cream <u>only on</u> <u>rare occasions</u> such as your birthday. Otherwise avoid them. Even though they may taste good, sugar is a known carcinogens.

√ Avoid sugar substitutes such as Saccharin, Splenda, Equal and others that may be carcinogenic. Use only Stevia as a sweetener— the only one that is natural and made from a plant.

√ Watch your glycemic index/load foods (those that raise blood sugar) because research shows a high glycemic load increases the risk of lung cancer compared to a low glycemic index/load diet. Avoid excessive servings or amounts of foods such as cakes, pies, candy, ice cream, bread, potatoes, muffins, pancakes, many cereals, and dates.

√ Many people are moving to a complete plant based diet that can be healthy and satisfying. If interested, you might consider trying it a couple days a week to start. You can supplement the fruit and vegetables, grain and nuts with juicing (below) and plant based protein powder drinks. Juicing allows you to absorb more fruit and vegetables that easily get to the cells and the powder allows you to get adequate protein that is often a concern of a vegan diet. Other deficits of a vegan diet may be vitamin B12, calcium, iron, zinc and Omega 3's., In 2016, The Academy of Nutrition and Dietetics warned of the risk of vitamin B12 deficiencies in vegans and vegetarians because they say they are found naturally only in animal products. This and other deficits of the vegan diet can be resolved with supplements, if necessary. See the expert interviews below.

√ More people are juicing regularly to obtain fresh juice that is quickly and easily available to the body cells in this form. If you haven't tried it, you might want to consider it as a step in the direction of better health. Use a variety of green and colored fruit and vegetables and experiment for the right taste. I add a granny smith apple or whole lemon including rind for the right taste. Juice should be consumed shortly after preparation for optimum benefit.

√Check your nutritional status periodically with the Nutritional Deficiency Test. Cancer patients, like the American public in general, tend to have nutritional deficiencies that may be a cancer causal factor. This is an important test that can identify deficiencies that can be corrected and assist in preventing cancer and other nutritional related diseases. Two of the laboratories that provide this test are **Spectrum Cell** Laboratories and **NutrEval** by Genova Diagnostics. The function of thirty-five nutritional components in white blood cells including vitamins, antioxidants, minerals, and amino-acids are evaluated by Spectra Cell. Research shows that testing the white blood cells gives the best picture of the bodies nutritional deficiencies. It also shows that deficiencies of vitamins, minerals, and anti-oxidants can affect the immune system and lead to degenerative diseases. Blood for testing can be drawn at your local lab or by your physician and mailed to Spectra Cell. A finder search engine for a provider near you is available on the site. Results show deficiencies in the body and provides recommendations for the needed supplementation. The thirty-five items are identified on their website at:

https://www.spectracell.com/patients/patient-micronutrient-testing/

NutrEval evaluates basically the same items as Spectra Cell and provides a 12 page report of results. See the sample here.

https://www.gdx.net/core/sample-reports/NutrEval_FMV-Sample-Report.pdf

More information on lab draws and so forth are in the link below. Reported costs of tests range from $1,000 to $1,800

https://www.gdx.net/product/nutreval-fmv-nutritional-test-blood-urine

Expert Interviews; Listen to several interviews on nutrition (plant-based, vegan, raw, organic, and other diets with some interviews related to cancer) and one interview on vitamins & antioxidants related to cancer and one on genetically modified organisms/foods (GMO's).

Dr Patrick Quillin PhD (beating cancer with nutrition) is an internationally recognized expert in the area of nutrition and cancer. He has 30 years' experience as a clinical nutritionist, of which 10 years were spent as the Vice President of Nutrition for Cancer Treatment Centers of America where he worked with thousands of cancer patients in a hospital setting. He has appeared on over 40 television and 250 radio shows nationwide and is a regular speaker for medical and trade conventions, including ACAM,

A4M, American Association of Naturopathic Physicians, and Integrative Medicine. He has been a consultant to the National Institutes of Health, U.S. Army Breast Cancer Research Group, Scripps Clinic, La Costa Spa, and United States Department of Agriculture; and taught college nutrition for 9 years. His 17 books have sold over 2 million copies and include the best sellers *Healing Nutrients* and *Beating Cancer with Nutrition* (Now translated into Japanese, Korean and Chinese) During the interview he tells us foods that will prevent or reverse cancer; common problems experienced by cancer patients and how nutrition can help these; supplements that cancer patients should take; ways to lower your cancer risk; and many other helpful tips. More information on Patrick can be found in the next link followed by our interview.

www.patrickquillin.com

https://www.holisticcancerfoundation.com/intervie ws-others-treat-related-health-concerns-cancer/

Dr Janice Strayer Ph.D (Plant Based Nutrition) is an author, educator, and health industry expert. Her mission in writing *The Perfect Formula Diet: How to Lose Weight and Get Healthy Now with Six Kinds of Whole Foods* is to help people and the planet through a whole foods, plant-based diet. Janice was motivated to research plant-based nutrition by the examples of her two daughters, who stopped eating meat at ages 11 and 13. She spent 14 years critically analyzing scientific findings until perfecting the whole foods discoveries she wants to share with you now. Janice has a Ph.D. in Human Development and Aging from University of California, San Francisco – one of the country's leading health sciences campuses. She is certified in plant-based nutrition through the T Colin Campbell Foundation and Cornell. She also has an M.B.A from University of California, Berkeley. More information is available at the next link followed by our interview.

http://www.perfectformuladiet.com

https://www.holisticcancerfoundation.com/intervie ws-others-treat-related-health-concerns-cancer/

Judy Scott (nutrition for anxiety) is a Food Mood Expert and Nutritionist, speaker and author of *The Antianxiety Food Solution: How the Foods You Eat Can Help You Calm Your Anxious Mind, Improve Your Mood & End Cravings*, published June 2011 by New Harbinger. Trudy has a nutrition practice with a focus on Food, Mood and Women's Health. She is President of the National Association of Nutrition Professionals and is a member of Alliance for Addiction Solutions and Anxiety Disorders Association of America. Trudy publishes an electronic newsletter entitled Food, Mood and Gal Stuff available at the next link followed by a link to our interview.

http://www.everywomanover29.comand http://www.antianxietyfoodsolution.com

https://www.holisticcancerfoundation.com/interviews-others-treat-related-health-concerns-cancer/

Susan Schenck (raw food coach) is a raw food coach and author of the 2 time award winning book *The Live Food Factor: The Comprehensive Guide to the Ultimate Diet for Body, Mind, and Spirit & Planet.* More information available at the next link followed by our interview.

http://www.rawguru.com/susan-schenck.html

https://www.holisticcancerfoundation.com/interviews-others-treat-related-health-concerns-cancer/

Andrea Beaman (Natural Foods Chef) is an author, and television host dedicated to alternative healing and green, sustainable living. Andrea was a featured contestant on Bravo's hit reality TV show, Top Chef (season 1). She is a regularly featured food and health expert on CBS News, and has appeared on Barbara Walters, The View, Emeril Live and Whole Living on Martha Stewart Radio. She is the host of the Award Nominated Fed UP! Andrea teaches fun cooking classes and health seminars to a wide base of clients and students at The Institute for Integrative Nutrition, the Natural Gourmet Cooking School, The James Beard House, The Open Center, and other schools around the country, to over 2000 students annually. She is the author of *The Whole Truth – How I Naturally Reclaimed My Health, and You Can Too* and *The Eating and Recipe Guide – Better Food, Better Health, and Health is Wealth – Make a Delicious Investment in You!*

She is featured in the Top Chef Cookbook, *Escape from Corporate America, Integrative Nutrition Case Histories and Louise Hay's Modern-Day Miracles.* She has contributed articles to Women's Health Magazine, Whole Living, Forbes Traveler, Dish Du Jour, Physician Assistant Magazine, Quick & Simple, Delicious Magazine, Nick Jr. Magazine, Delicious Living, and others. More information is available at the next link followed by the link to our interview.

http://www.AndreaBeaman.com

https://www.holisticcancerfoundation.com/intervie ws-others-treat-related-health-concerns-cancer/

Julie Daniluk (nutrition and inflammation) is the host of healthy gourmet on Own (Oprah Winfrey Network), and is a health expert for the Marilyn Denis Show (CTV) and has appeared on numerous TV and radio shows including the Dr Oz show, Lisa Live Radio, CTV's Breakfast, and TV/CP24's Wylde on Health. Television viewers will also recognize Julie from her busted segments on The Right Fit (OWN) where, acting as a nutrition encyclopedia, she examines the foods people need to stay healthy

She graduated from the Canadian School of Natural Nutrition, and becoming a cooperative owner of one of Canada's largest health food stores, the Big Carrot Natural Food Market, as well as health editor for Viva Magazine, a natural health publication with a circulation of over 120,000 coast-to-coast. She has spoken to parliament about the potential health risks of genetically modified food, and in order to bring food advocacy issues to a wider audience, Julie has been the event producer for Bio-Diversity with David Suzuki and Food share's Field to Table Festival. Her award-winning book, *Meals That Heal Inflammation* (Random House), is a #1 Amazon best-seller. More information is available at the next link followed by a link for our interview.

https://www.juliedaniluk.com/

https://www.holisticcancerfoundation.com/intervie ws-others-treat-related-health-concerns-cancer/

Marni Wasserman (plant based diet) is a Graduate of the Institute of Holistic Nutrition in Toronto and the Natural Gourmet Culinary School in New York, and is the founder of Marni Wasserman's Food Studio & Lifestyle Shop located in midtown Toronto where she teaches her signature cooking classes, and offers collaborative workshops and urban retreats. As a prominent figure of health and nutrition in Toronto, Marni is a regular contributor to Chatelaine, Huffington Post and Tonic Magazine. She made several TV appearances, been hosted on radio talk shows, consulted with The Windsor Arms Hotel for vegan and vegetarian menus, and participates in several live speaking and cooking demonstrations. She is also the author of the book *Plant Based Diet for Dummies*, *Fermenting for Dummie*s and several well-received plant-based eBooks. You can learn more about Marni by visiting her Facebook page, following her on Instagram, Twitter, or by checking her website in the next link followed by our interview.

www.marniwasserman.com.

https://www.holisticcancerfoundation.com/intervie ws-others-treat-related-health-concerns-cancer/

Jeffrey Smith (genetically modified foods) is an international bestselling author, award winning filmmaker, Executive Director of the Institute of Responsible Technology, and the leading spokesperson on the health dangers of GMO's. In 2012 Smith's feature-length documentary *Genetic Roulette, The Gamble of Our Lives* was awarded Movie of the Year (Solari Report) and (by Aware Guide) the Transformational Film of the Year. His books include: *Seeds of Deception: Exposing Industry and Government Lies about the Safety of the*

Genetically Engineered Foods You're Eating, the world's bestseller on GMOs, and *Genetic Roulette: The Documented Health Risks of Genetically Engineered Foods*, the authoritative work on GMO health dangers.

Mr. Smith has lectured in more than 40 countries, counseled leaders from every continent, and has been quoted by thousands of news outlets including: The New York Times, Washington Post, BBC World Service, The Times (London), the Associated Press, Reuters News Service, the LA Times, Time Magazine and the New Scientist. He appears frequently on radio and television on shows such as the Dr. Oz Show, The Daily Show with Jon Stewart, The Doctors, CBS News, Fox News, CNBC, NPR and Democracy Now. He is the founding executive director of The Institute for Responsible Technology (IRT) that is the most comprehensive source of GMO health risk information for consumers, policy makers, and healthcare professionals. More information in the next link followed by a link for our interview.

http://responsibletechnology.org/

https://www.holisticcancerfoundation.com/intervie ws-others-treat-related-health-concerns-cancer/

Dr. Kedar N. Prasad, (cancer and antioxidants) author of *Fighting Cancer with Vitamins and Antioxidants*, obtained a Master's degree in Zoology from the University of Bihar in India, a Ph.D. degree in Radiation Biology from the University of Iowa, Iowa City and Post-doctoral training from Brookhaven National Laboratory. Dr. Prasad joined the Department of Radiology at the University of Colorado Health Sciences Center where he became Professor in 1980. Later, he was appointed as the Director for the Center for Vitamins and Cancer Research. He has published over 200 papers in peer-reviewed journals including Nature, Science, and Proceedings of the National Academy of Sciences (PNAS). He has written several book chapters and abstracts as well as authored or edited 18 books on radiobiology, radiation protection and nutrition and cancer. He is a member of several professional organizations, and serves as an ad-hoc member of various Study Sections of the National Institute of Health (NIH). He is a frequently invited speaker at National and International meetings on nutrition and cancer. In 1982, he was invited by the Nobel Prize Committee to nominate a candidate for the Nobel Prize in Medicine. He was selected to deliver the 1999 Harold Harper Lecture at the meeting of the American College of Advancement of Medicine. He is a former President of the International Society for Nutrition and Cancer. Dr. Prasad has consistently obtained NIH grants for his research. His current interests are in the area of radiation protection, nutrition and cancer and nutrition and neurological diseases, particularly Alzheimer's disease and

Parkinson's disease. Since 2005, he is Chief Scientific Officer of Premier Micronutrient Corporation. More information is available at the next link followed by our interview link.

http://www.mypmcinside.com.

https://www.holisticcancerfoundation.com/intervie ws-others-treat-related-health-concerns-cancer/

₄2. D. Some Useful Supplements, Vitamins, Minerals and Herbs

(Many practitioners recommend getting vitamins and minerals from food, if possible, instead of relying on supplements, or avoiding supplements if you are in good health and have a good diet. Nothing is written in stone currently). Research presents conflicting findings on specific supplements and cancer causation/ prevention due to different dosages, length of time used, individual absorption, and other factors difficult to control in a research setting. Some tentative research findings are presented below for various supplements.

₄ ***Multivitamins.*** Research is contradictory on the relationship between cancer and multivitamins and minerals. Some research related to specific vitamins and cancer prevention follows with recommendations.

Beta carotene/vitamin A, One research study shows it protects the lungs against cancer producing toxins. Another study reported that ex-smokers who ate green and yellow vegetables high in beta carotene daily decreased their risk of stomach and lung cancer and a third study reported that beta carotene reverted precancerous breast cancer cells to normal cells. NB- when I had lung cancer in 1974 my doctor prescribed high dose beta carotene therapy for 1 years to revert precancerous cells to normal cells as part of my therapy. This practice was confirmed in the research above. By high dose I mean the following: I started with 200,000 IU daily for a week, then 100,000 IU daily for a week and then 50,000 IU daily for a year. (The recommended daily dose is 5,000 IU for this fat soluble vitamin) Because it can be toxic this should only be done under a naturopathic or other doctors care.

What to do:

> Eat orange and green vegetables such as carrots, sweet potatoes, spinach, kale, and other leafy green vegetables and if you do not get enough vitamin A consider taking a supplement.

Vitamin C: Research shows strong epidemiological evidence of a protective effect of vitamin C for non-hormonal-dependent cancers. In a review of 46 studies in which a dietary vitamin C index was calculated 33 found statistically significant protection with a high intake conferring a twofold protective effect compared to low vitamin C intake. Similar results were found in many additional studies using fruit high in vitamin C. Results showed protection against a variety of cancers including stomach, rectum, breast, cervix, lung cancer, esophagus, larynx, oral, and pancreatic. Several concluded that some ascorbic acid, carotenoid foods and other factors in fruit and vegetables act jointly to produce the results.

What to do:

√Increase fruits and vegetables in your diet, if needed.

Vitamin D3. Research is conflicting on vitamin D3 and cancer prevention. A current large study on colorectal cancer prevention and vitamin D3 will be completed in 2017. One study in 2011 reported 75% of all cancer patients had low vitamin D levels and those with the lowest levels had the most advanced cancers.

What to do:

√ Because of the above research physicians often recommend that patients with low vitamin D3 levels take high weekly doses of vitamin D for cancer prevention. Ask you physician for a 25-hydroxy vitamin D blood test to determine your level. Many insurance plans cover this.

√ If your level is low your doctor will prescribe a high weekly dosage to bring the level up to a normal level usually within 6 weeks.

√ Once you reach a normal level continue a daily supplement to maintain it, if necessary.

√ Get some sun daily, when possible, See discussion under ultraviolet rays above.

✤ Other Supplements/Herbs

Omega 3. According to the Cancer Research Institute Omega 3 may reduce cancer risk and also has cancer fighting properties.

What to do:

√ Fish such as salmon are recommended twice weekly.

√ If necessary take a fish oil supplement. Supplements should not be taken by those on blood thinners or with diabetics unless approved by your doctor.

Expert Interview: Listen to the interview with Dr Christopher Speed below on Omega 3. .

Dr Christopher Speed, MND, APO, is a tristate area based clinical nutritionist, dietitian, health expert and Director of Omega Wellness. He was the Food and Nutrition Strategist for Oldways Preservation and

Exchange, the first Global Director of Food and Nutrition Sciences at Ogilvy Public Relations Worldwide, founder of the North American chapter of Miami Nutrition USA, and sits on the Expert Panel at Mission Ready to help consumers realize the full extent to which omega-3's can support health and wellness. His major interest is Omega 3 and 6. His interview can be found at the following link:

https://www.holisticcancerfoundation.com/intervie ws-others-treat-related-health-concerns-cancer/

Probiotic. The American Institute for Cancer Research reported a study showing the value of probiotics in colon cancer prevention/ treatment but say further research is needed.

What to do:

√ American Institute for Cancer Research advises using probiotics, if desired, as a cancer preventive but make sure the product selected contains over 1 billion bacterium daily.

√ Continue other preventive activities such as exercise and nutrition.

Expert Interview: Board Certified Gastroenterologist **Lawrence Hoberman, MD,** is the creator of EndoMune Advanced Probiotic and founder of Medical Care Innovations. He has spent more than 40 years practicing medicine and is board certified in both

Internal Medicine and Gastroenterology. Frustrated by the lack of options to treat his patients suffering from Irritable Bowel Disease (IBD) in the early 2000s, Dr. Hoberman met with a PhD microbiologist to identify a combination of bacteria that might work to destroy the harmful bacteria living in the intestines, improving and maintaining the health of adults. The result is the development of his own effective probiotic supplement: EndoMune Advanced Probiotic. □Dr. Hoberman currently sees patients as a part of a health and wellness practice that stresses preventative medicine. He is in practice at Health by Design, located in San Antonio, Texas. He is available for speaking engagements about digestive health and the benefits of probiotics and has spoken at several conferences. More information is available at:

http://www.endomune.com

His interview follows:

https://www.holisticcancerfoundation.com/intervie ws-others-treat-related-health-concerns-cancer/

Garlic. Garlic may reduce the risk of certain cancers, has immune boosting properties, and suppresses growth of and fights certain cancer cells in the lab. It may also reduce the risk of prostate cancer, stomach and colorectal cancers and has many positive health benefits.

What to do:

√ Use garlic freely in cooking. It tastes great with vegetables, eggs and on bread.

√ Research/talk with your doctor before using if you are on a blood thinner for heart or other conditions. It thins blood and may cause bleeding.

Green Tea. Green tea contains polyphenols that are believed to have powerful anti-cancer properties. Preliminary research suggests a possible protective effect against bladder, esophageal, pancreatic, ovarian, and possibly cervical cancer, with as little as 3-5 cups a day. Evidence for breast, stomach, and lung cancer is mixed.

What to do:

√ Drink your tea daily as it is good for you.

√ If unable to consume tea consider taking a supplement for some protection.

Tumeric/Curcumin. Research shows some cancer prevention by using these supplements. In a clinical trial curcumin was given to 25 patients with pre-cancerous changes in different organs. This study showed that curcumin could stop the precancerous changes before becoming cancer. Another study showed lower rates of certain types of cancer in countries where people ate curcumin at levels of about 100 to 200 mg a day over long periods of time. In addition, several animal studies suggest that turmeric prevents colon, stomach, and skin cancers in rats exposed to carcinogens.

What to do:

√ Use some turmeric in your cooking.

√ Consider taking a supplement, if preferred.

√ Turmeric is a blood thinner so avoid it if you are taking warfarin or other thinners unless approved by your doctor.

√ There are many counter indications including some chemotherapy agents so check before using it if you have health issues.

42. E. Immune Builders

(Many people believe cancer occurs when there is a failure or compromise of the immune system which, holistically, occurs when there are multiple factors acting upon the human, agent, and environment triad discussed previously). Yet, despite the strong evidence for protection of a healthy immune system against bacteria, parasitic worms and virus, there is contradictory evidence on protection from cancer. However, Dr Corthay, a scientist from Norway presents evidence in favor of this theory. Some of his rationale includes: immunodeficiency in rats and humans associated with an increased cancer risk; organ transplant recipients treated with immunosuppressing drugs are more like to develop cancer; and those with immune deficiency due to HIV are at a higher risk of cancer. He continues to present 5 more convincing arguments for this connection.

What to do:

√It may be helpful to eat food or take supplements that will help maintain the immune system as a preventive action. There are different options available. Some are identified here.

√***Host defense***. A mushroom preparation called host defense-my community is made of 17 types of organically grown mushrooms. I have used these successfully for many years and used in combination with many of the other suggestions here I rarely experience health issues. I take 2 daily. Two well-known cancer clinics also used this product to build the immune system of cancer patients as part of their protocol. It can be purchase on Amazon or through a Google search.

√***Colostrum***. Some people, especially athletes, use colostrum as an immune builder but the research on its effect on the immune system is inconsistent, I used it periodically for several years but since it is made with bovine milk it is now inconsistent with my vegan diet. If selected you can use 6 capsules daily.

√***Beta-1,3d Glucan.*** This was recommended by Bill Henderson to stimulate the immune system. Avoid aspirin and NSAID while on this product. Available at http://ancient5.com

√***Enzymes.*** These have also been used to boost the immune system. As we age, we may experience stress, poor diet, environmental toxins and other challenges and as a result enzymes may become deficient in the body and supplementation may be necessary. Dr Steven Lamm on the Dr Oz show recommended taking the digestion test available for free at http://www.digesttest.com/ before selecting an enzyme. Symptoms of enzyme deficiency include gas, constipation, diarrhea, skin rashes, bloating, gastric upset and a lowered immune function. Enzymes are usually in pill form and may support the immune system of those who are gluten sensitivity, lactose intolerance, or support carbohydrates, fats, and protein digestion separately or in a blend of all. They are taken just before a meal to boost your own enzymes.

Expert Interview. **Dr Mark Moyad MD, MPH**, (He is involved in immune building, prostate and other cancer research and treatments.) He occupies an endowed position created and funded entirely by the patients he has helped over the past 15+ years as the Jenkins/Pokempner Director of Complementary and Alternative Medicine at the University of Michigan Medical Center (Department of Urology). He is also the primary author of over 130 published medical journal articles and is the former editor-in-chief of the medical journal *Seminars in Preventive & Alternative Medicine* by Elsevier. He is or has been an editor and reviewer for multiple diverse medical journals in Urology, Oncology and Alternative Medicine including most recently editor for the medical journal *Evidence-Based Complementary and Alternative Medicine*. Mark is the co-author or author of 9 books including his most recent *Dr. Moyad's No Bogus Science Health Advice: A step-by-step guide to what works & what is worthless, Beyond Hormonal Therapy-a guide for advanced prostate cancer patients*, and *Dr.Moyad's Guide to Male Sexual Health*.

Mark has maintained a consulting practice in Complementary and Alternative Medicine for the last 15+ years, and has lectured on breast, prostate and a variety of other cancers, cardiovascular disease and general health promotion internationally in almost every country and in all 50 states and at every major academic institution. He consults for and appears regularly in major magazines and television shows such as the Huffington Post, Fox News, the Dr Oz show, and Fitness magazine

Dr. Moyad has been active in the community and world and is the co-chair of the EAPPCa (Early Access Program for Prostate Cancer) committee, whose primary purpose is to negotiate and facilitate the delivery of ground breaking successful phase 3 medications to individuals with the most advanced forms of cancer while these medicines are in the 6-12 month window waiting for FDA approval. In 2013 Dr Moyad became part of the Promoting Wellness Foundation whose primary purpose is to improve access and the health and well-being of indigent patients around the world. More information is available at the following link followed by a link for an interview with him.

https://www.prostateconditions.org/about-pcec/council-members/34-mark-a-moyad-md-mph

https://www.holisticcancerfoundation.com/intervie ws-others-treat-related-health-concerns-cancer/

42. F. Sleep

(Sleep is important to maintain the immune system and prevent cancer). Research reports that the risk of cancer is higher if sleep is inadequate and/or disrupted such as while working nights. Read additional research on sleep on the cancer foundation website- under research on physical aspects→ other aspects→ sleep.

What to do:

√ Turn off televisions, computers, cell phones and other distractions an hour or two before bedtime to quiet the mind and prepare for sleep.

√ Avoid exercising, eating and drinking for several hours before sleeping.

√ Best to avoid caffeine drinks in the evening.

√A warm bath and a glass of warm milk before bed may be helpful. For those who do not drink milk, a cup of calming decaffeinated tea such as chamomile or lemon balm may help.

√Massage before bedtime, if available, is always helpful.

√Meditation and prayer before bedtime may help provide restful sleep.

√ Get from 7 to 8 hours of sleep nightly.

√ Infuse the sleeping room with lavender or Jasmin oil before sleeping.

Expert Interview −An interview with additional suggestions for sleep is available on the store page of the cancer foundation website. In addition to sleep suggestions it includes an additional hour of information on stress and stress management. Both by Dr Carl O Helvie.

≠2. G. Smoking Cessation

Cigarette smoke was discussed earlier under environment aspects of cancer prevention but because of its importance in cancer and other diseases and the effort needed by individuals to cease smoking it is repeated and enlarged upon here.

What to do:

√ Preparing to quit: 1) review your smoking history; 2) determine your nicotine reduction schedule (cold turkey, slow/fast reduction; 3) start a smoking diary; 4) learn/begin relaxation exercises; 5) start an exercise program a couple months before starting smoking cessation; 6) learn and use imagery such as imagining a place where you usually smoke and replacing it with you in the same place but drinking a glass of water, chewing gum, or drinking a calming herbal tea such as chamomile, peppermint, or lemon balm; 7) write a self-contract with positive and negative consequences of success or failure for every 7 days or 14 days such as giving up something or rewarding by a night out or dinner out. Also think about negative thoughts and ways to replace them with positive thoughts that are motivating such as replacing "I am more nervous since I quit smoking " with "I am aware of the changed mood since I quit smoking and I am replacing it with relaxation and imagery that make me feel better and healthier;": 8) find a support partner to utilize during the rough times, if possible; 9) establish a plan to visit family or friends during the first day of being smoke free for moral support; 10) determine your reason for quitting smoking that may be a strong motivating factor such as a reduced risk of cancer or heart disease; 11) decide the best way to quit-cold turkey, slow timed nicotine withdrawal, or with outside help; 12) research coenzyme Q10, vitamins and herbs that may be useful to correct smoke-related deficiencies such as vitamin C to protect against cell damage, vitamin B12 to improve liver function, or coenzyme Q10 to protect the heart and as an antioxidant to protect the cells.

√ Quitting 1) implement your smoking cessation plan; 2) review self-contract; 3) combine smoking cessation with a cleaning program that includes frequent bathing to remove toxins and frequent drinking of water to flush the system; 4) include the environment in the cleaning program by replacing filters in heating/cooling system, and cleaning the carpet, drapes, clothing and interior of your car; 5) implement or continue the exercise and relaxation programs, and use positive affirmations such as "I am happy to be a non-smoker," "My lungs are now clear and I can breathe easily" and "I am now healthy and happy;" 6) change your daily routine--on a sheet of paper identify triggers for smoking and replace these with new triggers such as replacing a thought of a cup of coffee with a cigarette with a new one of drinking a cup of tea or chewing a stick of gum and 7) watch your diet so you do not gain excessive weight.

Expert Interview: You can listen to an interview with **Dr Scott McIntosh** on smoking cessation on the following link (presented earlier) His biography was also presented under toxic chemicals.

https://www.holisticcancerfoundation.com/intervie ws-others-treat-related-health-concerns-cancer/

¢2. H. Sound (Music)

(A recent quote on Facebook by unknown—It is with your body that you dancer, but with your soul that you feel the music→ that recognized the interconnection of two parts of the mind-body-spirit triad. Thus, a reason why it is sometimes difficult to put a topic under one overall category instead of another). Research shows music can help reduce pain and stress; can improve coping, mood and a sense of wellbeing; lower heart rate, blood pressure, and breathing rate; and can relieve chemo induced nausea and vomiting. Read additional research under research→ mental/spiritual aspects→ sound/music research and cancer on the cancer foundation website. .

What to do:

√ Listen to classical, meditation or other soothing music regularly.

√ Avoid rock, and rap music or any music that is unpleasant to you.

√ Sing in a church choir, if desired. Research shows that 1 hour weekly will decrease stress hormones and increase protein in the immune system.

Expert Interviews: Listen to interviews on sound (music) and healing below.

Sharon Carne, BMus, M.F.A. (sound healer) is an author, speaker, musician, recording artist, sound healer, Reiki master and consultant. She has been a faculty member of The Conservatory at Mount Royal University in Calgary, Alberta since 1988. Sharon is the founder of Sound Wellness, whose programs are at the forefront of education in how sound and music can be easily applied to your everyday life – to reduce stress, help you concentrate, energize you, support your health, bring harmony to your life and so much more. Sharon is the author of *Listen from the Inside Out,* and has produced and recorded several CDs, solo and with others. She is invited to speak about sound healing to a wide variety of corporate and private audiences, many within the medical community. More information is available at the next link followed by our interview.

http://soundwellness.com/

http://holisticcancerfoundation.com/interviews-mental-spiritual-aspects/

Joseph Carringer (didgeridoo music and healing) is a professional didgeridoo musician and sound therapist who uses concert class didgeridoos, combining Traditional Chinese Medicine meridian and organ theory with Ayurvedic Chakra philosophies creating a unique and powerful therapeutic sound, music and healing experience. Joseph has been playing an

Australian Aboriginal didgeridoo for over 15 years, using it as a deep meditative tool. He performs both nationally and internationally on mind/body connection and the effects of didgeridoo sound therapy for the purposes of clearing energetic and emotional stagnation within the energetic body. Since the fall of 2005, Joseph has offered yearly classes for the Maine Medical CAM programs and the University of Southern Maine's CAM programs, and presents at the University of New Hampshire and New England College. He also volunteered music and healing at Maine Medical Center, Portland, ME on R-1 (cardiac) and Pediatric floor.☐Joseph has been on John Holland's Hay House Radio and a guest speaker at John's Chakra-Healing class at Kripalu Center for Yoga presenting his Didgeridoo Chakra Clearing Workshop. It is Joseph's goal to help people realign their bodies' natural rhythms on a cellular level through harmonic therapy. He has a variety of CD's for sale. More information is available at: http://www.didgetherapy.com/

Our interview is available at:

http://holisticcancerfoundation.com/interviews-mental-spiritual-aspects/

Dr. Carrol McLaughlin is an award-winning professor, heading one of the largest and most respected harp departments in the world. She is a renowned concert harpist who performs internationally as a soloist and with orchestras. Carrol has given workshops and lectures in more than 30 countries, teaching performers to overcome fear and achieve at their highest potential. An expert in Neuro Linguistic Programming, a Kundalini yoga teacher, an author, and a composer, Carrol is also a gifted healer. She has recently conducted a study at the University of Arizona Medical Center, researching the power of harp music to heal patients in the intensive care unit following heart surgery. She is also the author of *Manifesting Moment to Moment.* More information is available at the next link followed by our interview.

http://music.arizona.edu/faculty_staff/profile?netid=c mclaugh

http://holisticcancerfoundation.com/interviews-mental-spiritual-aspects/

Jonathan Goldman (music, sound healing) is an international authority on sound healing and a pioneer in the field of harmonics. He has worked with masters of sound from both the scientific and the spiritual traditions and has been empowered by the Chant Master of the Dalai Lama's Drepung Loseling Monastery to teach Tibetan Overtone Chanting. Jonathan is author of *Healing Sounds, Shifting Frequencies: The Lost Chord,* and *Tantra of Sounds:*

Frequencies of Healing that was coauthored with his wife Andi. He was winner of the 2006 Visionary Award for "Best Alternative Health Book" for his best-selling *The Seven Secrets of Sound Healing*. He is Director of the Sound Healers Association and President of Spirit Music, Inc in Boulder, Colorado. A Grammy nominee, Jonathan has created numerous best-selling, award winning recordings including The Divine Name with Greg Braden in 2012: AscensVisionary Award, a Grammy nominee in Harmonics and Chakra Chants that was a double winner of Visionary Awards for "Best Healing Meditation Album" and "Album of the Year," He is a lecturing member of the International Society for Music Medicine and has dedicated his life to the path of service, helping awaken and empower others with the use of sound to heal and transform. He presents Healing Sound lectures, workshops and seminars worldwide. More information is available below followed by our interview.

www.healingsounds.com

http://holisticcancerfoundation.com/interviews-mental-spiritual-aspects

Part 3. Individual Factors-Mental/Spiritual Aspects

On the Holistic Cancer Foundation website you will find research on the relationship of mental/spiritual interventions and cancer prevention, and can listen to the interviews with Dr Lise Alschuler, Dr Francisco Contreras, Dr Veronique, Dr Gawler and interviews with several survivors (especially Dr. Carl O. Helvie) who all use a holistic approach to cancer prevention/treatment including mental/spiritual interventions in addition to physical interventions. These combined components (physical, mental, spiritual) form a holistic approach and are more effective that physical interventions alone. Some mental/spiritual interventions for preventing cancer or reducing potential causal symptoms are presented below.

43. A. Affirmations

(Affirmations have been used effectively for many years to improve self-concept, lose weight, gain friends, obtain a new job, place to live, and/or other individual needs). Although there is little research on the value of affirmations for cancer, there is limited research that shows affirmation improve memory, and reduce blood pressure, heart and breathing rates. Dr Anne Marie Evers used affirmations to reduce the effect of chemo symptoms during her cancer journey and wrote about this to help others who choose chemotherapy for their cancer intervention.

What to do:

√ Use affirmations or positive thoughts to counteract negative thoughts. For example, instead of saying "I feel so alone because I have no friend." Say" I am a wonderful person who has many friends."

√ Affirmations should always be present oriented starting with "I am" or "I have" statements instead of future oriented ones starting with "I will have" or "I want". Future oriented affirmations are never attainable because our mind will keep them out of reach.

√ Some affirmations may be useful for you to start a change process. Examples include "I am healthy and happy at my ideal weight." "I am at the ideal weight for me" or "I am attractive at the ideal weight I have obtained." Or I am at the right size and weight for me" if you want to lose weight; or "I have a wonderful fulfilling job" or "I have a wonderful boss and co-workers who support and respect me" for those who want to improve relations in their job; or "I am a wonderful person who has many friends" or "I am a loving person surrounded by love" for those wanting more friends. One that my friend

Dr Evers told me recently is "I am 1% healthier (or 2% or 5% or any other number) today than I was yesterday." You might also say "I am happy and healthy and free of cancer and other diseases." If you doubt the potential effectiveness of using affirmations as part of a preventive regime read about epigenetics and the amazing effect of thoughts on our genes.

Expert Interview: listen to interviews with two experts on affirmations below.

Dr. Anne Marie Evers is a Best Selling Author of many books on the power of Affirmations. She is an Ordained Minister and Doctor of Divinity. She is co-author of *Wake Up and Live the Life you Love in Spirit* with Dr. Deepak Chopra and Dr. Wayne Dyer. Dr. Evers is an International Motivational Speaker and Talk Show Host. Her popular book, *Affirmations: Your Passport to Happiness* is in its 6th printing. She has created the popular Cards of Life. Dr. Evers has been teaching the power of affirmations and helping people for many years and she believes that when properly done, they always work! Her recently published book, following her experience with cancer and chemotherapy, was written to help others and discusses her using affirmations to reduce the side effects of chemotherapy. The book *70 Ways to Cope with Chemo* with a foreword by Dr Bernie Siegel is available at Amazon. More information is available at http://www.AnneMarieEvers.com

My interview with Dr Evers follows.

http://holisticcancerfoundation.com/interviews-mental-spiritual-aspects/

Dr Patricia Crane talks about how she first discovered the power of affirmations; how listeners can use principles to create affirmations; why affirmations do not always work; how she cured herself with chronic fatigue syndrome with affirmations and other holistic interventions; and the difference between affirmations and visualization. Dr Crane is a protégé of Louise Hay and has worked with her for 22 years. More information is available at:

http://www.selfgrowth.com/experts/patricia_crane.html

Our interview follows.

http://holisticcancerfoundation.com/interviews-mental-spiritual-aspects/

♦3. B. Compassion

(Compassion has been defined as the emotional response when perceiving suffering and involves an authentic desire to help). Research shows that expressing compassion increases DHEA, a hormone that reverses aging, by 100% and decreases cortisol, the stress hormone, by 23%. It also increases your happiness and the happiness of others around you. It has been identified as one of the main tools for developing happiness. In a study with cancer patient's the compassion of health professionals reduced anxiety in cancer patients. For additional research see research on the cancer foundation website at research→ mental/spiritual aspects→ then under compassion.

What to do: the following will help you develop this important spiritual attribute. (You will note that many spiritual practices here have similar components and you may be able to combine some of them or work on some one week and different ones another week).

√ Start each day with happy thoughts. The Dalai Lama offers an affirmation that may be helpful. "Today I am fortunate to have woken up, I am alive, I have a precious human life, and I am not going to waste it. I am going to use all my energies to develop myself, to expand my heart out to others, to achieve enlightenment for the benefit of all beings, I am going to have kind thoughts towards others, I am not going to get angry or think badly about others, I am going to benefit others as much as I can."

√ After you become comfortable with the above you may develop your own affirmations using the guidelines presented under affirmations earlier. One might go as follows: "It is a wonderful day-I am alive, rested, and have lots of energy for which I am thankful. I will be aware of others today and will have kind thought for them. I will avoid getting angry and will be understanding of those who disagree with me. I will accept things as they happen and will thank God for the many opportunities."

√ Look for things you have in common with others such as a need for love, a need for food and shelter, and a need for attention and happiness. After reflecting on commonalities in general you could go through a list of common needs you share with others you meet in day to day life. Think mentally to yourself just like me, this person is seeking love and happiness. Just like me this person is trying to avoid suffering and humiliation. Just like me, this person is seeking to fulfill his/her needs. Just like me, this person has felt sadness, loneliness and despair.

√ Empathy is an important part of compassion and can be learned using visualization. Visualize daily a loved one suffering pain as a result of an accident or some other terrible situation. I think of a movie I watched a few days ago called Snow Bound in which a young couple with a baby were stuck on a road in a snow storm many miles from any houses or a community and how they were forced to walk miles before finding help and the aftermath of frostbite on their feet, partial amputations, dehydration, malnutrition and other painful experiences. Visualize the suffering in as much detail as possible. After a couple weeks visualize someone else you know beyond your loved ones and repeat the above process. At a later time you might also consider a prayer box in which you place the names of all who request prayers and pray for all of them daily. I have a few hundred names in my prayer box and hold the box during meditation every evening. At the end of my meditation I pray for the group in the prayer box and channel energy from my meditation to them. In closing I ask for the best for all and add "For the good of all parties concerned."

√ After you can visualize suffering of others reverse roles and visualize you going through the suffering. Visualize how much you want that suffering to end. Then visualize another person wanting your suffering to end and does something to end it. Feel the happiness and joy of their support and comfort and open your heart to that person. Reflect on any feelings you have. Obtaining this feeling will grow with practice. After you become good at visualizing these roles do something small for another person each day such as running an errand, doing a chore, smiling at a stranger, or listening to their problems. After you become good at this make it a part of your daily routine and later expand your good acts throughout the day to those who mistreated you or who you mistreated. Reflect on someone you mistreated and who reacted with kindness, Visualize your responded to that person and replay the experience with a more positive feelings and emotions that you might use next time. Use this as a model for future behavior so that you slowly react with kindness when mistreated by another.

√ At the end of each day take a few minutes to review the day including the people you met and talked with, and how you interacted with each other. Did you act with compassion? Could you improve your practice? How? Can you use the improved practice the next time you encounter similar situations. Congratulate yourself.

Expert Interview: Listen to the interview with Simon Fox below.

Simon Fox, Executive Director of the Adventures in Caring Foundation (AiC), is co-Author of *What Can I Say? A Guide to Visiting Friends and Family Who Are Ill* and co-producer of five video-based training programs on compassion including *The Medicine of Compassion* and *Oxygen for Caregivers*. For 30 years AiC has taught the art and practice of compassion—as a skill that restores well-being and promotes healing. It was founded by Simon's wife, Karen Fox, in 1984, and the nonprofit is most famous for its Raggedy Ann and Andy volunteers who visit local nursing homes and hospitals to lift the spirits of patients who are lonely. The Adventures in Caring team has decoded and now teach undergraduate students from the University of California–Santa Barbara who are studying to become doctors, nurses, and allied health professionals in a one-year service-learning internship. After in-depth training they visit the residents in a nursing home or the patients on a hospital unit on a weekly basis for a school year.

More than one thousand hospitals, one thousand hospices, two thousand churches, and several hundred nursing schools have used AiC's programs. Santa Barbara City College School of Nursing has integrated the entire AiC Cultivating Compassion series into its new Memory Caregiver program that teaches nursing assistants how to build better relationships with patients who have dementia. Visiting Nurse and Hospice Care of Santa Barbara has trained its own team of mentors to teach the Cultivating Compassion program throughout the entire agency, to equip its staff with the most advanced skills for communicating compassion to the sick and dying. Even the American Trauma Society in Washington DC used AiC expertise—to help teach trauma surgeons how to better communicate with the families of trauma victims in those crucial moments when they must deliver news right after surgery. For more information, visit:

www.AdventuresInCaring.org

Our interview follows.

https://www.holisticcancerfoundation.com/intervie ws-mental-spiritual-aspects/

₄3. C. Faith

(Faith is the "confident assurance that something we want is going to happen". According to the living bible "it is the certainty that what we hope for is waiting for us, even though we cannot see it up ahead". Faith cannot be learned by reading about it. It must be used with positive results). For research on faith go to research→ mental/spiritual aspects→ faith and prayer.

What to do:

> √ Because faith is the opposite of doubt, worry, and fear start with a situation in which this occurred in your life. 1) Bring the situation to mind such as fear of loss of a job, a significant relationship, money worries, or other concerns. 2) Relive the experience including feeling the emotions. 3) Next replace the negative feeling with faith or knowing that God will bring only the best to you. 4) Would you have faith in a similar situation in the future?

√ Make a list of all experiences in which you used faith. 2) Analyze the factors that influenced your faith at those times. 3) How did you feel after the experiences were over? 4) Have you repeated the use of faith in similar situations?

√ Look at your past and find situations in which you did not use faith. 2) Relive one experience. 3) Replace the lack of faith with faith in the situation. 4) How would you react in a similar situation in the future?

√ Over the next week be consciously aware of situations in which doubt and fear creep into your thoughts. 2) Immediately replace the thought with knowing that God is looking out for you and will bring only the best to you. Whatever happens is for your greatest good and ultimate happiness. 3) Were you successful in replacing negative with positive thoughts? 4) How did you feel? 5) You are beginning to experience faith. Pat yourself on the back.

√ Sometimes when we worry and become self-centered in our thoughts we become isolated and that reinforces the negative feelings. At such times the following may help: 1) think about what interests you such as politics, helping sick people, helping the elderly, developing spiritually, or getting in physical shape, 2) select one area of interest and get involved: join a political action group, volunteer for meals on wheels, in a nursing home, or a hospital, join a faith community, spiritual group, or optimistic group such as the Association for Research and Enlightenment study group, or Optimist Club, or join Weight Watchers, as appropriate.

Expert Interviews: Listen to interviews with experts on faith and healing below.

Dr Harold Koenig, M.D., M.HSc, completed his undergraduate education at Stanford University, his medical training at the University of California at San Francisco and his geriatric medicine, psychiatry, and biostatistics training at Duke University. He is board certified in general psychiatry, geriatric psychiatry and geriatric medicine, and is on the faculty at Duke University as Professor of Psychiatry and Behavioral Sciences, and Associate Professor of Medicine. He is also a registered nurse (R.N.). Dr Koenig is founder and former director of Duke University's Center for the Study of Religion, Spirituality and Health, and is founding Co-Director of the Current Center for Spirituality, Theology and Health at Duke University Medical Center. He has published extensively in the fields of mental health, geriatrics, and religion, with close to 350 scientific peer-reviewed articles and book chapters and nearly 40 books in print or in preparation. He is the former editor-in-chief of the *International Journal of Psychiatry in Medicine* and of *Science and Theology News*. His research on religion, health and ethical issues in medicine has been featured on over 50 national and international TV news programs (including the Today Show, ABC's World News Tonight, and several times on Good Morning America), over 100 national or international radio programs (including multiple NPR and BBC interviews), and hundreds of national and international newspapers and magazines (including cover stories for *Reader's Digest, Parade Magazine, and Newsweek*). Dr Koenig has given testimony before the U.S. Senate (September, 1998) and the U.S. House of Representatives (September 2008) concerning the effects of religious involvement on public health. He has been interviewed by James Dobson on Focus on the Family and by Robert Schuller in the Crystal Cathedral on the Hour of Prayer. He has also been nominated twice for the Templeton Prize for Progress in Religion. Dr Koenig's latest books include *The Healing Power of Faith* (Simon & Schuster, 2001), *The Handbook of Religion and Health* (Oxford University Press, 2001:2011 forthcoming), his autobiography, *The Healing Connection* (2004), *Faith and Mental Health* (2005), *In the Wake of Disaster* (Templeton Press), *Spirituality in Patient Care, 2nd Edition* (2007), and *Medicine, Religion and Health* ((2008) published by Templeton

Foundation Press. Dr Koenig travels extensively to give workshops and seminar presentations. More information is available at the following link followed by our interview. :

https://spiritualityandhealth.duke.edu/index.php/harold-g-koenig-m-d

https://www.holisticcancerfoundation.com/intervie ws-mental-spiritual-aspects/

Radhanath Swami is a Vaishnava Sanyassin (a monk in a Krishna-bhakti lineage) and teacher of the devotional path of Bhakti-yoga. He is author of *The Journey Home*, a memoir of his search for spiritual truth. His teachings draw from the sacred texts of India such as *The Bhagavad-Gita*, *Srimad Bhagavatam*, and *Ramayana*, and aim to reveal the practical application of the sacred traditions, while focusing on the shared essence which unites apparently disparate religious or spiritual paths.

Born Richard Slavin, on December 7, 1950, in his teens he came to confront a deep sense of alienation from suburban Chicago life and the civil injustices of mid-century America. At the age of nineteen, while on a summer trip to Europe, his internal struggles culminated in a commitment to search for God wherever it might lead him. In Vrindavan he found the teacher he was searching for in A.C. Bhakti Vedanta

Swami Prabhupada (1896-1977) the founder of the International Society for Krishna Consciousness (ISKCON), and a representative of Gaudiya Vaishnavism, (the Krishna-bhakti tradition stemming from the 16th century mystic avatar Sri Chaitanya). In choosing Bhakti Vedanta Swami, as his guru, Radhanath Swami felt compelled to shear his matted locks and reenter Western society with a mission to share the sacred wisdom he had received. This return exemplifies the form of devotional yoga which is at the heart of Radhanath Swami's teachings, a spiritual practice expressed as tangible action meant to bring about personal fulfillment and benefit the world.At the age of 31 he took the monastic vows of a Vaishnava Sanyassin and became known as Radhanath Swami. Today Radhanath Swami travels regularly throughout India, Europe and North America, sharing the teachings of Bhakti-yoga. He resides much of the year at the Radha Gopinath Ashram in Chowpatty, Mumbai. For the past twenty-five years he has guided the community's development and has directed a number of acclaimed social action projects including Midday Meals, which daily serves more than 260,000 plates of sanctified vegetarian food to the children of the slums of Mumbai. He has also worked to establish missionary hospitals and eye camps, eco-friendly farms, schools and ashrams, an orphanage, and a number of emergency relief programs throughout India.

More information available at the next link followed by our interview.

http://www.radhanathswami.com/

https://www.holisticcancerfoundation.com/interviews-mental-spiritual-aspects/

The following **3 expert interviewees** all practiced faith in their recovery from illnesses.

Debbie Campanelli is very compassionate and always ready to help others. She is a leukemia survivor who was told she was terminal in 1976 and subsequently was cured by her faith in Jesus. Her story has been confirmed by articles in medical journals and in the National Inquirer. If you are fortunate you will meet her on Facebook. A link to our interview follows.

https://www.holisticcancerfoundation.com/interviews-cancer-survivors/

Mary McManus has known challenges since she was five years old beginning with contracting paralytic polio and then enduring nine years of violence at the hands of family members. But those early challenges helped her to grow into the woman that she is today. Paralytic polio and trauma made Mary stronger. She has a fiery Spirit and moves forward undeterred by the challenges she faces in life. In 2007 after receiving the diagnosis of post-polio syndrome, a "progressive neuromuscular disease" by Western Medicine standards, she took a leap of faith leaving her award winning almost 20 year career as a social worker at the Department of Veterans Affairs to heal her life. She discovered the gift of poetry in her soul. Her pen became her divining rod for healing as she put a call out to the Universe to imagine herself healthy, whole, and free, running unencumbered and reclaiming her life from the thieves in the night who tried to take life away from her. She landed right smack in the middle of the glorious life she leads today. When Mary was told she would not and could not run again after a knee injury in December of 2014, she was blessed to find her way to Jeffrey Spratt, MT who pioneered the Spratt Method of Muscular Therapy, He is also the Owner and Principal of Spratt Muscular Therapies, LLC, an innovative massage therapy practice that was the game changer for Mary in her healing journey. Through the power of positive touch, Mary healed the effects of paralytic polio and trauma and is now going the distance on the roads and in her life. Mary's philosophy is that we can go the distance whatever the challenge and whatever goals we set. Partnering with Spratt Muscular Therapies, LLC Mary reclaimed her life and reclaimed her advantage. She went on to run the 2016 Bermuda Half Marathon that had been on her bucket list for 3 years. Mary came out of retirement to work for Jeffrey and Spratt Muscular Therapies as his

Communications and Public Relations Director. More information available at the next link followed by our interview.

http://marymcmanus.com/

https://www.holisticcancerfoundation.com/interviews-mental-spiritual-aspects/

Richard Schooping Inspirational Author, Speaker, Volunteer, and Singer who transcended AIDS and is now helping others live fearless, balanced, and empowered lives. He published his journey in *From Suffering to Soaring Through God I Transcended AIDs*. More information at the next link followed by our interview.

http://www.richardschooping.com/

https://www.holisticcancerfoundation.com/interviews-mental-spiritual-aspects/

43. D. Forgiveness

(Many unforgiving individuals have anger and hatred feelings that create chronic anxiety that in turn produce excess adrenaline and cortisol. These excesses deplete killer cell production needed by the body to fight disease. Some cancer hospitals have begun offering support groups for those who are unable to forgive.) Research reports that people who forgive are more likely to have higher self-esteem, lower blood pressure, fewer stress-related health issues and better immune system function, among other health benefits. Sixty one percent of all cancer patients have forgiveness issues and 50% of these are severe according to Dr Michael Barry, pastor, and author of *the Forgiveness Project.*

What to do:

√ Sit quietly with your eyes closed. Use the following affirmation: the individual I need to forgive is_____, and I forgive him/her for _____. Say this over and over. Then imagine the person saying to you "I set you free and I forgive you and thank you for your kindness." Do this for 5 or 10 minutes at a session. Repeat this process for each person and each transgression in your mind. After you finish search for the experiences you have harbored and release them.

√ Sit quietly in a meditative state. Think of the person you believe has harmed you. Visualize him/her and say "I forgive you for not being the way I want you to be. I forgive you and I set you free." (Hay, 1984) You will feel a burden lighten from your heart and chest.

√ Forgiving yourself is also important. Repeat over and over for a few minutes the following "I forgive myself for _____. It may be necessary to use the affirmations to forgive self and others over a number of days or weeks until a new pattern has evolved.

Hay, Louise (1984) *You Can Heal Your Life*. Hay House.

<u>Expert Interview</u> Listen to the interview with **Dr Frederic Luskin, PhD**, who is Director of the Stanford University Forgiveness Project, Director of Wellness Education at Stanford University, and Professor of Clinical Psychology at Sofia University. He is author of *Stress Free for Good*, *Forgive for Good*, and *Forgive for Love*, and *Forgive for Good: A Proven Prescription for Health and Happiness* (2002) He is renowned for teaching about the psychological and medical benefits of forgiveness. Research done by Luskin and others has confirmed that forgiveness can reduce anger, depression, and stress while it leads to greater feelings of optimism, hope, compassion, and self-confidence.

As director of the Stanford University Forgiveness Project, Luskin conducts an ongoing series of workshops and research projects that investigate the effectiveness of his forgiveness methods on a variety of populations. The forgiveness project has explored forgiveness therapy with people who suffered from the violence in Northern Ireland and Sierra Leone, as well as from the attacks on the World Trade Center

September 11, 2001. In addition, his work has been successfully applied and researched in corporate, medical, legal, and religious settings. His work has been featured in Time; O, The Oprah Magazine; Ladies' Home Journal; US News & World Report; Parade; Prevention; the New York Times; the Los Angeles Times; the Chicago Tribune; USA Today; and the Wall Street Journal. Luskin is also a professor at the Institute of Transpersonal Psychology. He offers lectures, workshops, seminars, and training nationwide on forgiveness, stress management, and emotional competence. More information is available at the following link followed by our interview.

http://greatergood.berkeley.edu/author/fred_luskin

http://holisticcancerfoundation.com/interviews-mental-spiritual-aspects/

43. E. Gratitude

(Gratitude has been defined as the quality of being thankful, or a readiness to show appreciation for and to return kindness. The best way to benefit from gratitude is to notice new things you're grateful for every day). Recent research reports that people who practice gratitude regularly have stronger immune systems, lower blood pressure, and fewer symptoms of illness. They generally sleep better and can also better tolerate their aches and pains. Gratitude encourages resilience after difficult experiences, strengthens relationships and promotes forgiveness. Read some additional research on the Cancer Foundation website under research→ mental/spiritual→ gratitude.

What to do:

√ Keep a gratitude journal. Write things that you are grateful for daily or weekly.

√ Reflect regularly on how the things you are grateful for are often taken for granted or how life would be different if they were not present.

√ When you are unhappy or stressed review and reflect upon your grateful entries to help the brain revert to a grateful mode.

√ When you wake up in the morning use one or two grateful affirmations such as *I am grateful for this beautiful sunny day* to start your day.

√ Be mindful of things as they occur that make your day brighter such as a beautiful sunset or a chance encounter and discussion with a friend. This reflection facilitates mindfulness of the good around you.

√ Periodically think of others who brought good into your life and consider the effort they made to do that. Perhaps they spent time purchasing a gift, or saved time for you in a busy schedule, Confirm your gratefulness for these people in your life mentally or by a telephone call, email message, or note to say hello. Expressing gratitude is important so thank others in your daily interaction, when appropriate.

√ Find positive quotes that express the power of gratitude and share with others such as on Facebook or Twitter. I have several friends who do this and it is something I am grateful for.

√ Use prayers of gratitude daily to acknowledge the good things in your life. I find this the most important aspect of gratitude. .

Expert Interview: Listen to **Dr Phil Watkins** who received his B.S. in psychology from the University of Oregon and his Ph.D. from Louisiana State University. He has taught in the Psychology Department at Eastern Washington University since 1990. After investigating memory biases in depression, Phil shifted his focus to gratitude and how it impacts well-being. He developed one of the most utilized measures of gratitude (the GRAT), and has been called a "pioneer in gratitude research." He has remained active in the science of gratitude, and his current research focuses on how gratitude enhances happiness. He has published a number of scientific papers on gratitude, and has also published two books. His first book, *Gratitude and the Good Life*, is a treatise on the current science of gratitude. More recently he published *Positive Psychology 101*, which is written for a more general audience on the science of happiness and positive psychology (Springer Publishers, New York). More information available about Phil in the link below followed by our interview.

http://greatergood.berkeley.edu/author/Phil_Watkins

http://holisticcancerfoundation.com/interviews-mental-spiritual-aspects/

₄3. F. Meditation

(Meditation for me is blanking the mind so that God can speak with us. It differs from prayer in which we speak with God. There are several types of meditation and I have followed the Cayce method for almost 50 years.) Much research on meditation over many years shows results for cancer patients including improved quality of life; reduced stress, depression, tiredness; being more positive and optimistic; improved sleep, and reduction of chronic pain among other effects. For additional research go to the research tab→ mental/spiritual tab→ then meditation.

What to do:

√ Preparing for meditation varies from person to person. You may choose to cleanse the body with soap and water. Some people eat certain foods before meditation or a light meal. Some do a series of deep breathing (Edgar Cayce recommends #3 brief relaxation below). Some do a series of head and neck exercises before deep breathing. In these, you sit straight in a chair. Close your eyes. Drop the head forward and return to normal position 3 times. Then drop it backwards and return to normal position 3 times. Then repeat to the left three times and to the right three times. Then roll the head in a circular pattern from left to right three times, and then right to left three times. Some people have recently been concerned about rolling the head too far back and thus, move it in a more horizontal position as they move it back and forth. However, I continue to roll it as before.

√ Some people like sound and smell as part of the process. You may choose to listen to Gregorian chants or meditation music and also burn incense such as Sandalwood during the process.

√ Some people like to meditate alone and others prefer to meditate with groups. A couple good groups to meditate with are Edgar Cayce Search for God groups that can be found worldwide, or a traditional Friends (Quaker) silent church service where members meditate until the spirit moves them to speak. Edgar Cayce groups can be located by emailing the address on their website http://www.edgarcayce.org/ or calling toll free 800-333-4499, or 757-428-3588 and ask for the study group office.

√ The process of meditation also varies. There are many types of meditation but I present the meditation process advocated by Edgar Cayce. Sit quietly-preferably in the same place at the same time each day. Clear the mind of usual thoughts such as today's daily activities or those planned for tomorrow. Focus on an affirmation or phrase from the bible such as "Not my will, but thine, O lord." In the *Search for God* book used by study group members there are affirmations for each chapter being studied on such bible passages as above. Empty your mind of all thought and as your mind wanders come back to the affirmation and again blank your mind. Continue this process for at least 20 minutes. Over time you will find that it becomes easier to sit, clear your mind, and listen for God.

Expert Interviews: Listen to the following interviews on meditation with experts.

Dr Leslie Phillips: is a speaker, author, workshop leader, meditation teacher, healer and clairvoyant reader. She is passionate about the benefits of meditation and has taught 1000's of individuals and has spoken at 100's of events. Her book *The Midas Tree* is a spiritual adventure novel that contains the secret to life, and is enjoyed by adults and kids everywhere. Her Portico Card Deck is used by many to activate their intuitive abilities. During her training in metaphysics and spirituality at the CDM Spiritual Teaching Center, she was mentored by renowned author and speaker Mary Ellen Flora. She graduated as an ordained minister from their Clairvoyant Training Program in 2003 and from the centers teaching program as a meditation and healing teacher in 2005. Before going to Canada in 1998 Dr. Lesley was also trained in meditation, healing and clairvoyance at the School of Insight and Intuition, Richmond UK. Prior to that she was a member of The Rainbow Bridge Dream Work Group where she explored dream incubation, dream re-entry, astral travel, shamanic journeying, and dream symbol interpretation and has kept a dream diary since childhood. More information is available at the next link followed by the link to our interview.

http://drlesleyphillips.com/

https://www.holisticcancerfoundation.com/interviews-mental-spiritual-aspects/

Padma is one of Canada's best known teacher of meditation and yoga. She writes and hosts a daily national TV series called Living Yoga with Padma. She studied meditation in the Himalayas of India for 8 years; mastered Sanskrit text of philosophy and is authorized to teach meditation and yoga by the director of the International Meditation Institute of India. Padma was director of the Padma Yoga and Meditation Center in Vancouver, B.C. and currently leads courses and workshops there. She holds a B.Sc. degree in Biology from McGill University, Canada. More information is available in the next link followed by our interview.

http://www.padmayoga.ca/

https://www.holisticcancerfoundation.com/intervie ws-mental-spiritual-aspects/

43. G. Optimism/Positive Attitude-Behavior

(Optimism has been defined as hopefulness and confidence about the future. Because of the difficulty in separating the concepts of optimism and being positive, they are combined here). In a research study cancer patients defined positive attitude as optimism for the day and getting though everyday events of the journey by taking control rather than focusing on the future. Research on optimism has been shown to increase health and prevent illnesses, is inversely related to distress, increases the quality of life and longevity of cancer patients, and decreases the cancer antigen (ca125) which shows improvement. Additional research studies may be found at the Cancer Foundation website under research→ mental/spiritual aspects→ optimism.

<u>What to do:</u>

√ Practice gratitude discussed above because it helps you focus on being more positive and optimistic.

√ View your life as a journey in which you look forward to new experiences and are optimistic about those experiences.

√ Spend 5 minutes each morning thinking positive thoughts about the upcoming day including the people and events that will bring you happiness. What parts of the day will be most enjoyable? What do you look forward to? Carry this optimism with you throughout the day.

√ Each evening write in an optimistic journal about 2 or 3 good things that happened during the day.

√ Surround yourself with optimistic people that you meet in person or interact with on Facebook, LinkedIn or other social media. Be influenced by these and other positive people. When faced with negative situations talk with someone you trust and ask/receive honest feedback.

√ Remove or discourage negative people in your life either those you meet in person or on social media such as Facebook. Recently I had to remove the fifth negative person (non-friend) on Facebook in many years so in general they are few for which I am happy.

√ Reduce or eliminate your reading about or listening to the news or other media programs/articles that may have a negative influence on you. I do not have television in my house and have not seen a movie at the theatre for over 25 years. I spend my free time reading or watching movies from the 30's, 40's, or 50's when there was less sex, violence, and controversy in them.

√ In general, pay attention to the old saying "Avoid discussing politics and/or religion." This can influence your emotions in a negative way unless your discussions are with others of a like mind. When I visit my sister over Christmas there is a rule that there will be no discussions of politics and that is a good one because of the differing views and emotions engendered.

√ Fill you mind with so many positive thoughts there is no room for negative ones. When you wake up in the morning say to yourself "What a wonderful day—I feel so great today—I look forward to being together with my colleagues" and other positive thoughts. Repeat these and other positive thoughts through-out the day. If you have a negative thought immediately replace it with a positive one. For example, when someone cuts in front of you while driving to work, mentally bless them, and wish them a great and SAFE day.

√ Affirmations discussed earlier may assist in remaining positive and optimistic.

√ If you have a recurring negative thought or feeling such as fear of flying you can try the following. Do this exercise for 3 to 7 days until the negative feelings stops. Close your eyes. Choose a stressful situation such as the fear of flying. Bring the thought to your attention. Imagine a situation in which it could occur such as when you are flying. Interrupt the though by snapping your fingers, repeating the word stop, or setting off an alarm., replace the negative thought or feeling with a positive one such as visualizing yourself flying and looking out the window at a beautiful mountain or lake.

√ Listen to uplifting music. Or if you can sing, try that. It can also be uplifting and according to research it has positive effects on you. I remember when my mother was alive and living upstate New York, I always sang the last hundred miles of driving because I was so happy for the opportunity to see her, and there was minimal traffic and beautiful mountains and valleys to look at. I also search Facebook for uplifting music and share that on my page. I replay it often and read the positive comments from friends.

√ Do something nice for someone else to take attention off your own problems. You will feel good about what you do.

Read positive quotes. I always look for these on Facebook and share them on my page. I go back and review them periodically and look at comments from other positive people.

Interview I have no interviews at present but will add to the website and newsletter when available.

⁴3. H. Prayer

(In her book, *Dreams Your Magic Mirror*, Elsie Sechrist said meditation does not lessen the need for prayer, because it does not take the place of prayer. Prayer is a mental activity on our part addressed to God. Meditation is a listening state so that we may hear God speak to us. Prayer comes before meditation, before the affirmation; and we may pray, if need be, all day long as we go about our daily work. Jesus found it necessary at times to pray for long periods. Certainly prayers should be a constant activity of the religious heart). Research shows that people who pray live healthier lives, are sick less often, recover faster, are less often depressed, and have a lower death rate from cancer and heart disease. Read further research on prayer under research→ mental/spiritual aspects→ faith, prayer and cancer research on the Cancer Foundation website. There are two types of prayers: prayers for self and prayers for others. Some prayer practices are discussed below.

<u>What to do:</u>

√ There are four types of prayers that should be used often: petition, thanksgiving, praise, and confessional.

√ Some people think prayers are asking for something. This type of prayer (petition) is the most used prayer, and involves asking for what we want such as a new house, improved health, resolving a problem in a relationship, a new position, and other wants. Jesus said ask and you shall receive and I believe all prayers are answered. However, it may not be answered within your time frame and by the time it is answered you may have moved on to something else you want. Receiving what we ask for may also depend upon how deeply we want it. It also must be in our best interest. In my prayers of petition I always end with "If it be thy will, O Lord. Bring only the best to me and others."

√ A second type of prayers is prayers of thanksgiving. This involves expressing gratitude to God for what we have and for what he has provided. When we are thankful in our lives, we develop an attitude of gratitude and become more content with what we have. This keeps our mind filled with positive thoughts and away from the negative ones. These prayers also build faith. You should offer prayers of thanksgiving daily and may be thankful for your health, your home, friends, job, food, family, weather, spiritual awakening or whatever is appropriate in your life. Gratitude that is widely discussed now is closely related to prayers of thanksgiving.

√ A third type of prayer is praise that involves giving honor and devotion to God for who he is. It means putting God first above all others and is an automatic response to awe and amazement. It can be in the form of singing (Psalms 9:2, 149:1; Mark 14:26); verbal praise (Psalm 103:1); lifting up of the hands (Psalm 63:4, and 134:2); clapping (Psalm 42:1); kneeling (95:6); bowing (95:6) or with music (Psalm 150:3-5).

√ The final type of prayer is confessional and may mean asking for forgiveness for wrongdoing, or recognizing and articulating to God your feelings, attitudes, and problems.

These prayers allow you to feel God's acceptance and support.

√ If you have a problem with another person or dislike someone try the following. 1) Pray for that person daily for one week. Pray for his/her health and prosperity and the best in life for him/her. 2) After one week evaluate how you feel about him/her. Often it will seem like the person has changed but usually you have changed in your feelings toward him/her. And as you change your feelings and attitudes you will move to a higher level of consciousness that will be reflected in your interactions with him/her and he/she will react to your changed actions in a different way. This outcome has a positive effect on your health because the anger, resentment or other negative emotions are gone.

√ It may be helpful to do some of the preparatory exercises prior to prayer that were mentioned under meditation. These include; head and neck exercises, deep breathing, relaxation exercises, incense, if desired, and background music. I prefer having my healing session following meditation when the energy has built up and can be sent to others who need it and/or have requested it. Like meditation I pick the same time and place daily for prayer.

√ Try the following: 1) Pray at the same time daily for one week. 2) Try including the four types of prayer identified. 3) After one week evaluate any changes that have occurred. 4) Ask yourself: Do you have more energy? Do you feel happier and more optimistic? Are you less incline to worry or have negative feelings?

√ A second prayer session for one week could focus on the following. 1) Identify a problem that you have been concerned about. 2) During daily prayer ask for guidance from the higher self/being. 3) Whenever you think of the problem during the week, think a positive thought or use a positive affirmation. 4) Evaluate any changes in your attitude toward the problem or movement toward solution of the problem after one week. .

Expert Interviews: I do not currently have interviews focusing specifically on prayer but you can listen to about 12 interviews that include prayer under interviews→ mental/spiritual interventions→ faith, love, balance, and spiritual healing on the Holistic Cancer Foundation website that includes Dr Harold Koenig and others or under faith above. .

https://www.holisticcancerfoundation.com/intervie ws-mental-spiritual-aspects/

43. I. Relaxation Exercises

(Different authors include different practices in relaxation exercises/techniques. For example, Cancer Care includes deep breathing, meditation, and visualization under relaxation techniques. I separate meditation, and visualization from exercises and may include breathing.) Research shows that relaxation exercises may reduce anxiety and increase comfort levels of cancer patients. Other research showed it reduces stress, headache and insomnia. Research studies on relaxation exercises and health/cancer can be found at: the cancer foundation website under research tab→ mental/spiritual aspects→ relaxation exercises.

What to do:

√ Brief relaxation 1 exercises. Carry these out 3 times a day. Sit comfortably in a chair and close your eyes. Concentrate on remembering the most peaceful setting you have been in. This might be sitting on a mountain overlooking a quiet village, sitting by a pond watching ducks swim by, or fishing in a river in an isolated setting. With each breath think to yourself relax, relax. With practice, your worries will float away.

√ Brief relaxation 2 exercises. -Carry these out 3 times a day. Close your eyes. Inhale deeply through the nose, hold, then exhale through the mouth. While exhaling mentally say the word "peace" or "one."

√ Brief relaxation 3- close your eyes. Breathe in deeply through your left nostril and exhale through the right (you will need to hold one nostril with your finger). Next breath in through the right nostril, and exhale through the left. Next breath in through the nose (both nostrils) and exhale through the mouth. Repeat 3 times.

√ Progressive relaxation- relaxes 15 to 20 major muscle groups from your feet to your head. Sit or lie in a comfortable position and loosen clothing, if necessary. Close your eyes. Concentrate on your breathing and be aware of breathing in and out. Say the words "in and out" while breathing, if not distracting. When you are calm, begin instructing your muscle groups to relax. Begin by thinking "feet relax, feet relax." Then "calves relax, calves relax." And "legs relax, legs relax." Continue up the body until you finish the neck and head. Then again focus on your breathing. Do some deep breathing as before. Now you are ready to sit up or stand up and should feel relaxed.

√ A variation of this is as follows. Do this once a day. Tense each muscle hard for 7 to 10 seconds, but do not strain, and visualize the muscle group, if desired. Relax the muscle group abruptly and relax the muscle for 15 to 20 seconds letting them go completely limp. You may repeat the phrase "I am relaxed" as you relax the muscle, if desired. Repeat the muscle relaxing and tensing for each muscle group.

43. J. Serving Others

President Monson of the Church of the Latter Day Saints said "I believe that love is shown by how you live, how you serve, and how you bless others. When we serve others, we are showing them that we love them, and we are also showing Jesus Christ that we love Him." I believe when serving others we benefit more than the person being served because God has given us a wonderful opportunity to help another human being.

Although I believe motivation to help others is an important part of cancer prevention and recovery I found little research on this. However, the American Psychological Association notes that research to answer why people volunteer and additional research in other related areas of serving others is forthcoming. Possibly the lack of research is because it overlaps with spiritual attributes of gratitude, and compassion that are included here and that may be easier to study. When I do find research I will be back to work further on this section. There are many ways to help others and some will be identified below. You will think of many others.

What to do:

√ Provide transportation when needed. For example, I live alone and when I need a medical procedure such as minor surgery or a hospital procedure where I cannot drive afterwards there are a couple neighbors I know who will take me, wait, and bring me home. This support means a great deal to me.

√ Find time to talk with others and help them resolve issues, if appropriate. I know a waitress who always has time to talk with customers and many return week after week for this interaction.

√ Invite someone to dinner or take dinner to a shut in neighbor.

√ Volunteer for Meals on Wheels or for serving meals at a homeless shelter. A friend in Florida told me today she was filling in for someone who was sick and was enjoying the experience with Meals on Wheels.

√ Provide assistance to someone stranded on the highway. Several years ago my brother and his family broke down on their way to visit me in Virginia-this was before cell phones, I phones etc. Someone stopped and helped them resolve the issue so they could continue on their way. My family were so grateful for the assistance.

√ Cut grass or shovel snow for an elderly or house bound neighbor. A few years ago I went by rescue squad to the hospital. At about 8 p.m. they discharged me from the emergency unit but there were no buses, taxis, or other means of transportation moving because of a snow storm. I finally reached a neighbor who came to pick me up and also shoveled my drive way when we got home. What a relief this was to me over the next few days while the snow remained on the ground and I could easily get to the mailbox. .

√ Take baked goods to work or to a community or organizational affair.

√Talk with people at parties who seem uncomfortable or out of place.

√ Pay for a strangers coffee in line behind you. This has become a popular concept recently.

<u>Expert Interview</u>: Listen to the interview with **Simon Fox** under compassion again as he and his wife run a volunteer organization that provides clowns to cheer up hospital patients and he discusses the benefits of helping others. Although an important part of curing or staying healthy (I believe) I do not have an interview

currently on serving/helping others but will add one when I find the right person.

#3. K. Social Support/Isolation

(A support system is one of three components of successfully resolving a crises situation in a healthy way. From personal experience it is also important when an individual is initially facing a diagnosis of cancer.) **A**lthough there is not convincing research evidence of a relationship between social support/ isolation and the development of cancer there is evidence of a relationship between social support/ isolation and the progression of cancer. Thus, it is important to develop a support system when healthy (during the primary prevention phase of health). Additional research under research→ mental/spiritual aspects→ social support/isolation on the Holistic Cancer Foundation website.

 What to do:

> √ A support system begins with building relationships and the most important of these is with yourself because you cannot love or care for another until you care for yourself. Learning to love one's self is a long complex process but a simple way to start is to look at yourself in the mirror and repeat, I *love you (your first name) just as you are.* Repeat several times each session and several times throughout the day.

Repeat this process daily until you feel the effect. You might also use *I approve of myself. I approve of myself* and repeat several times daily. There are many helpful books to improve your self-esteem but one I like is *You Can Heal Your Life* by Louise Hay who discusses the above process. .

√ If you want to establish relationships with others assess your areas of interest and find clubs or organizations in your community that match those. Then join and become involved.

√ You might also attend classes or workshops that interest you at the local university or other appropriate organizations in order to meet people of like mind.

√ Join a church or spiritual/positive group such as the *Edgar Cayce Search for God Group* or the *Optimist Club*.

√ If you need to focus consciously on building/maintaining relationships with others try the following: 1) mark your calendar or appointment book with special days such as birthdays and anniversaries of family and friends and acknowledge/celebrate those days with them.

√ Establish a goal of meeting and talking with one new neighbor, club member, church member, or other person each week.

√ Join at least one new organization or club of interest each year.

√ On a regular basis send a note or email to a friend just to say hello.

√ Invite a friend to dinner at least monthly.

√ Share problems and successes with family and friends regularly.

√ Acknowledge births, deaths, anniversaries, birthdays and other special occasions with cards or phone calls.

√ Call elderly or disabled friends/neighbors regularly and offer assistance.

√ Volunteer at local organizations such as Meals on Wheels or a homeless shelter at least once a month.

43. L. Stress Reduction/Management

(There are multiple aspects to stress causation requiring a holistic approach for long term management.) Research shows contradictory results for a relationship between stress and cancer but a strong link between chronic stress and cancer progression and metastasis. Thus, it is important to develop techniques to reduce stress in one's life. Find research studies on stress and cancer at: research→ mental/spiritual aspects→ stress and cancer on the cancer foundation website. Many of the holistic things to do to reduce or eliminate stress offered below are long term processes that take time to learn but are worth the effort.

What to do:

√ Eat an alkaline diet that will reduce acid reflux and other physical stress situations in the body. Edgar Cayce suggested an alkaline diet comprised of 80% alkaline producing foods and 20% acid producing foods. Alkaline producing foods include fruit, vegetables and milk products (for those who use dairy products). Acid producing foods include meat, grains, and sweets. See the discussion earlier under nutrition and alkaline diets.

√ In stressful situations walk around the block or count to 10 before reacting.

√ Obtain adequate sleep and rest. Seven to eight hours of sleep are recommended.

√ Do regular relaxation exercises (discussed earlier).

√ Learn visualization techniques and use them as needed.

√ Work on changing your attitude from negative to positive. For example, if someone cuts in front of you when you are driving, wish them well and say a little prayer that they will arrive safely instead of a more usual verbal response or physical gesture. You will find that as you become more positive the driving experience becomes more enjoyable. Use this approach in all aspects of your daily activities for a relatively stress free life.

√ Use affirmations (discussed earlier) to help stay positive and stress free.

√ Pray for others who are difficult. If you pray for someone who is difficult for a week you will believe he/she has changed. However, it may be you who has changed and as you changes the other person changes to accommodate the new changing you. As you become more positive, he/she becomes more positive and there is less stress.

√ Develop spiritual attributes such as forgiveness and faith (discusses previously).

Expert Interview Listen to the interviews on stress and stress management below.

Dr Kathy Gruver is an award-winning author and the host of the national TV show based on her first book, *The Alternative Medicine Cabinet* (winner Beverly Hills Book Awards). She earned her PhD in Natural Health and has authored two books on stress: *Body/Mind Therapies for the Bodyworker* and, *Conquer Your Stress with Mind/Body Techniques* (Winner Indie Excellence Awards, Beverly Hills Book Awards, and Finalist for the USA Best Books Award). She has studied mind/body medicine at the famed Benson-Henry Institute for Mind-Body Medicine at Harvard Medical School and pursued further education at The National Institutes of Health. Gruver has been featured as an expert in numerous publications including Glamour, Time, Wall Street Journal, CNN, WebMD, Prevention, Men's Health, Huffington Post, Yahoo.com, Ladies Home Journal, Massage and Bodyworks Magazine, and Massage Magazine. She has written dozens of health and wellness articles and contributing posts. Dr. Gruver has appeared as a guest expert on over 200 radio and TV shows including NPR, Sky News London, CBS Radio, and Lifetime Television, and has done over 100 educational lectures around the country. For fun and stress relief Dr. Gruver does flying trapeze and hip hop dance. A recent winner of NAWBO's Spirit of Entrepreneurship Awards and nominee for the Gutsy Gal Awards, Kathy maintains a massage and natural health practice in Santa Barbara, Calif., also offering phone and email health consultations. She has also produced an instructional massage DVD, *Therapeutic Massage at Home; Learn to Rub People the RIGHT Way™* and is a practitioner with over 20 years of experience. Her award-winning book, *The Alternative Medicine Cabinet* was recently turned into a national talk show. More information can be found at the following link followed by our interview.

www.thealternativemedicinecabinet.com.

https://www.holisticcancerfoundation.com/intervie ws-mental-spiritual-aspects/

Paul Huljick: Chairman and Joint CEO, co-founded Best Corporation, a pioneering organic foods company listed on the stock exchange. While leading the company during which its value grew to more than $100 million, he eventually developed a number of severe stress-related conditions and was diagnosed in 1998 as suffering from bipolar disorder as a result of years of unchecked stress, When he experienced a nervous breakdown Huljick was informed that there was no cure and that he would inevitably relapse. Determined to free himself of his conditions, he began a comprehensive search for answers and ultimately succeeded in mastering his stress, overcoming his conditions and achieving a healthy, positive way of life by developing and implementing his nine-step overall wellness plan that is discussed in *Stress*

Pandemic: The Lifestyle Solution, 9 Natural Steps to Survive, Master Stress and Live Well (July 31, 2012, Mwella Publishing).

He has been featured in *Psychology Today* "One of this seasons most talked about books", *Publishers Weekly* "valuable resource", *Forward Magazine* "awareness and prevention can be a powerful tools for wellness", *Kirkus* "A commonsense guide to managing everyday stress, *"reviewed by the American Institute of Stress as* "well researched and scientifically proven" *and* interviewed by more than 180 radio shows nationwide including BBC and CBS. Huljick had numerous television appearances including Fox25 and Fox5 and was featured in more than 140 newspapers and magazines. Paul presented on a 20 Stress city book tour ending in a seminar on "say 'No' to stress" in Maui – Hawaii. He wrote Stress *Pandemic* while in New York. More information is available at the following link followed by our interview.

http://www.StressPandemic.com

https://www.holisticcancerfoundation.com/intervie ws-mental-spiritual-aspects/

A presentation on stress and stress reduction/ management and sleep on a CD by **Dr Carl O Helvie** is available in the store on the Holistic Cancer Foundation website.

♣3. M. Visualization

(There are two types of visualization-process and outcome. Process visualization involved imagining in detain each of the action steps needed to obtain the desired outcome or goal, and outcome visualization involves envisioning yourself obtaining the desired outcome or goal in great detain using all of your senses. In reality they are best used together for overcoming illnesses or stress situations and obtaining what you want in life. Research shows visualization works because neurons in our brains, (electrically charged cells that transmit information) cannot distinguish between imagery and real life and thus, interpret imagery as a real-life action. When we visualize an action, the brain generates an impulse that tells our neurons to "perform" the movement. This creates a new neural pathway causing our body to act in a way consistent to what we imagined. Thus, without actually performing the physical activity your body achieves a similar result.) Research shows that visualization can help alleviate nausea and vomiting from chemotherapy, extend life, mobilize the immune system and reduce pain of cancer patients, and helps patients obtain other goals. Further research can be found at: research→ mental/spiritual aspects→ visualization on the cancer foundation website.

What to do:

√The following process outcome visualization exercise should be practiced three times a day for 10 to 15 minutes. It has been used for such conditions as anxiety, asthma, headaches, viral infections, pain reduction, and enhancing the quality of life. It works well with affirmations. 1) Close your eyes. 2) Imagine the illness or stress and visualize it in any way you prefer. For example, you may see cancer cells as black blobs in your arteries, a headache as marbles rattling around in your head, or viruses as jelly in your arteries. 3) Picture treatment in your mind and see it eliminating the attackers or strengthening your body. For example, treatment may be visualized as increasing the number of knights on horseback that attack, kill and carry the dead cells away or the treatment may be visualized as white cells that eat the jelly and clean the arteries; it may be visualized as pushing the marbles out of the head by way of the nose or mouth, or it may be visualized as receiving healing from God or some other higher being as you visualize his laying his hands on you. Treatment may also be imagined as a cool throat and warm chest for chest congestion, peace and love for anger, or coolness in hot areas. 4) Imagine the body free of pain and healthy. 5) Pat yourself on the back and tell yourself that you have done a good job of eliminating the condition.

√ Practice daily for five minutes and use your imagination to see yourself as successful, having the relationship you want, closing an important deal, crossing the finish line at a race, owning your dream house, getting an A on an exam, remaining healthy, overcoming a headache or whatever you wish to manifest. Always imagine you already have the outcome you wish for (see affirmation process). Do not hope for something or imagine one day you will have it but instead imagine you already have it because out subconscious mind cannot distinguish between what is real and what is imagined and if you visualize something as happening in the future it will always remain in the future. For example, if you want an A on an exam, imagine yourself looking at the grade sheet and seeing an A by your name, feeling the excitement of the event, seeing yourself calling your parents with the news, seeing yourself celebrating with friends and smelling and eating your favorite food, or other images appropriate to the event.

√ It works best to combine the two types of visualization and use them with appropriate affirmations.

Expert Interview: see Interviews with 4 experts below. In addition, read about epigenetics.

Laurel Clark, D.M., D.D., is a teacher with the School of Metaphysics, a past president of that organization, and the Vice President of the International Association for the Study of Dreams. She is also an interfaith minister, counselor and author. She speaks frequently about dreams, visualization, and developing intuition to educational institutions, professional organizations, and businesses. Her most popular books are *Intuitive Dreaming, The Law of Attraction and Other Secrets of Visualization, Dharma: Finding Your Soul's Purpose*, and *Karmic Healing*. More information is available at the following link and then a link to our interview. :

http://som.org/board-of-directors/laurel-clark-d-m-d-d/

https://www.holisticcancerfoundation.com/intervie ws-mental-spiritual-aspects/

Sara Carapizzi. Sara has worked in yoga for 15 years and is currently Director of the School of Royal Yoga in Chester, New Jersey. More information can be found at the following link and our interview beyond that.

http://www.theroyalpathwaysinc.com

**https://www.holisticcancerfoundation.com/intervie
ws-mental-spiritual-aspects/**

Pamela Harper, R.N., is best known for her ability to combine BODY, MIND & SPIRIT to facilitate healing by treating the whole being no matter what else is happening. Renowned speaker on the subjects of "Health, Wealth and Life Purpose" she is a number one best- selling author, media personality, psychiatric registered nurse, success coach, counselor and hypnotherapist. Many of her admirers attribute their personal accomplishments to her ability to get to the source of their problems and offer immediate solutions. "Right Here, Right Now" using a combination of ancient wisdom is her motto. Pamela has a private practice in Irvine, CA and treats individuals who are looking to create more immediate results. A link to more information follows and the interview is after that.

http://therapycable.com/TC/business-
directory/1211/pamela-harper/

**https://www.holisticcancerfoundation.com/intervie
ws-mental-spiritual-aspects/**

Michelle Beaudry, CHt, is a fulltime clinical hypnotist in the Orlando, Florida area; and a member of the National Guild of Hypnotists, Hypnosis Education Association, and Conscious

Awareness Network. More information available in the following link followed by our interview.

https://trans4mind.com/counterpoint/index-spiritual/baudry.shtml

https://www.holisticcancerfoundation.com/intervie ws-mental-spiritual-aspects/

43. N. Pre-Cancer Testing and Lifestyle Changes for Prevention

Introduction: Some exciting new tests that identify biochemical changes associated with cancer and that may eventually lead to cancer if not corrected have been developed. These tests offer the opportunity to make lifestyle changes to reduce cancer risk or the severity of cancer long before it occurs.

AMAS - Anti-malignin antibody screen test
This test is designed to pick up cancers before the patient has other signs and symptoms, and months before conventional medical tests can detect it. The test is good for early stage cancers but for advanced cancer, if the anti-malignin antibody is wiped out, the test doesn't work. Reports on the test are contradictory but in one study of over 8,000 patients the test was 95% accurate in detecting cancer. Oncolab will send a free test kit for you to take to your doctor. The test runs about $150 in addition to your doctor's office

charges for drawing blood. Call 1-800-9CATest for a test kit and information

The CA Profile Test is a test for early cancer detection with an 87 to 97% accuracy. It is based upon the assumption that there are detectable biochemical changes that occur in the human body prior to but during its transformation into a cancerous state. It is known that cancer evolves over many years as a renegade cancer cell develops into a cancer tumor. Some of the processes that occur during tumor development can be measured such as the C-reactive protein and the fibrinogen that indicates chronic inflammation. Chronic insulin resistance, high cholesterol levels and weakened immune functioning also contribute to a weakened body resistance. In addition, the gradual buildup of chemical toxins and heavy metals in the body may contribute to the mutational changes seen in aberrant cancer cell growth. And last unresolvable chronic stress may be the final burden to the body's defenses.

The Cancer Profile is comprised of the following 8 tests.

- HCG is human chorionic gonadotropin, which is tested under 3 different methodologists, serum chemiluminescence assay and immunoradiometric assay, and urine quantitative chemiluminescence assay,

- PHI is phosphohexose isomerase enzyme,
- CEA is carcinoembryonic antigen,
- GGTP is gamma-glutamyltranspeptidase,
- TSH is thyroid-stimulating hormone),
- DHEA-S is dehydroepiandrosterone sulfate)

Dr Emil Schandl, who developed the test after many years of reading, testing, and experimenting at the Howard Hughes Research Institute and local hospitals in Miami, has seen markers elevated in patients as many as 10 to 12 years before diagnosis of cancer. Knowing the time necessary to develop cancer allows individuals diagnosed by the test to make lifestyle changes to hopefully prevent or reduce the effect of cancer. In addition, the test is useful for clinical laboratory follow up and monitoring disease reduction or progression.

While each test included in the Profile might not be indicative enough when analyzed alone, together they provide an impressive level of accuracy. "Looking at three cancer markers together (HCG, PHI, CEA), 221 positives in 240 breast cancer patients (92 percent) were detected. Of lung cancer patients, 127 of 129 (97 percent) were correctly diagnosed. And with colon cancer patients, 55 positives out of 59 patients (93 percent) were correctly identified." "Also included in the profile are the DHEA-S, TSH, and GGTP tests. These are peripherally related to cancer. The rationale is that people with either low thyroid activity, low adrenal activity, or abnormal GGTP results seem to be predisposed to cancer." More information is available at the following link.

https://www.americanmetaboliclaboratories.net/ca-profile.html

Although the above site does not identify price for the test, it is listed as $300 at the Mind Body Medicine Center website https://www.healmindbody.com/the-ca-profile-a-new-test-to-detect-cancer

The ONCOblot test (Ecto-Nicotinamide Adenine Dinucleotide Oxidase Disulfide-Thiol Exchanger 2 or (ENOX2) is another test for early cancer detection that identifies a specific type of protein in the blood, ENOX2, that exists only on the surface of a malignant cancer cell. The protein is shed into the circulation, can be detected in the blood, and is a highly sensitive marker for the confirmation of cancer. It can be detected as early as stage 0 or when there is 2 mm or less of tumor mass that is about the size of a pinhead (estimated 2 million cells) compared to several billion cells needed for a positive mammogram. Thus, it can be detected before it is visible on any scans or other tests. It can also determine which organ it is growing in.

Over 200 articles have been published in Scientific Journals on the test and its database contains the following 25+ ENOX2 transcript variants:

• Bladder • Breast • Cervical • Colorectal • Endometrial • Esophageal • Gastric • Hepatocellular • Kidney • Leukemia • Non-Small cell • Lung Small cell • Lymphoma • Melanoma • Mesothelioma • Myeloma • Ovarian • Pancreatic • Prostate • Sarcoma • Squamous Cell • Follicular Thyroid • Papillary Thyroid • Testicular Germ Cell • Uterine.

Tests will be positive for Stage 1 and Stage 4 disease, and stage 4 recurrence disease but not in the blood of non-cancer (healthy) volunteers, nor in survivors who were free of disease for 1 to 5 years.

The test can be used in combination with other tests such as a high PSA, abnormal mammogram, or suspicious PET scan. It also confirms biopsy results and detects cancer in high risk populations. It can also be used to confirm post treatment effectiveness.

In early 2016 the cost of the test ranged from $850 to $1,000. The Reno Integrative Medical Center charges $1,000 for the test. However, in 2016 one newspaper in Canada listed the price as $1700. The ONCOblot lab will only send the kit to your physician who draws the blood and returns it to the lab. Results are sent to your doctor and usually take 3 weeks. Plans are underway to obtain insurance coverage. More information is available at: http://oncoblotlabs.com/

Goals of the Carl O. Helvie Holistic Cancer Foundation

Obtain and provide funds for research on holistic medical/health care as a means of curing cancer and increasing the quality of life;

Provide patient education on the use of holistic medical/health information as a form of prevention and cancer treatment;

Provide financial/other assistance to those in need of holistic care in the treatment of cancer, if funding is available.

Support research and education on environmental toxins that cause cancer or other medical ailments;

Bring awareness to the state and national legislatures regarding the use of holistic medical/health care as a recognized and scientifically based form of prevention and treatment of cancer.

Biography of Dr. Carl O. Helvie

Carl O. Helvie, R.N., Dr.P.H. completed his basic nursing education and passed his national certification for registered nurse in 1954, He completed his baccalaureate in nursing (BSN) from New York University in 1958, his master's in public health nursing (MS) from the University of California (San Francisco) in 1961, his master's in public health (MPH) in 1966 and his doctorate in public health (Dr.P.H.) in 1969 both from Johns Hopkins University, School of Public Health.

He has over 60 years of experience as a nurse practitioner, educator, author, and researcher including staff positions at the Monroe County Hospital, Rochester, New York, and the V.A. Hospital in San Francisco, California, and a staff and head nurse position at Bellevue Hospital in New York City. He was a staff public health nurse at the Oakland and San Francisco Health Departments in California. He later held teaching positions at the University of California (San Francisco), Duke University (Durham, North Carolina), Old Dominion University (Norfolk, Virginia) and the University of Applied Sciences (Frankfurt, Germany). He has been host of the Holistic Health Show on BBS Radio since 2008.

Dr Helvie has published 9 books and chapters in 4 additional ones and has published over 100 scientific articles or research papers presented internationally. He worked with colleagues in Germany, England, Russia, Czech Republic, Spain, and Denmark on research, publications, and presentations about homeless populations and on home care. Over a 35 year period he developed and refined the *Helvie Energy Theory of Nursing and Health* that is used internationally in at least 9 countries. He also established and administered a nursing center that provided primary health care for homeless and low income individuals and families using one of his federal grants for over $800,000. He has been recognized in most major references such as Who's Who in Virginia, Who's Who in American Nursing, Outstanding Educator in America, and American Men and Women of Science. In 1999, he received the Distinguished Career in Public Health Award from his peers at the American Public Health Association. He also has 2 listings on *Wikipedia*.

Dr Helvie is also a 44-year lung cancer survivor who was given 6 months to live by traditional medicine and subsequently used holistic all natural interventions to overcome cancer. Continuing with a modified holistic lifestyle following recovery he avoided a recurrence of cancer and also arrived at age 85 without chronic diseases or prescribed medications until recently. He has been interviewed on over 150 radio and television shows around the United States and Canada for his last two books and has given papers on lung cancer at several conferences nationally. In addition, he was interviewed for over 40 magazine articles. In 2014 he founded and is President of the Carl O Helvie Holistic Cancer Foundation. Because of his continuing activities in holistic health since 1970 while serving as a volunteer summer camp nurse for the Edgar Cayce Association he has been called a pioneer in holistic health and nursing. More information is available at:

www.HolisticHealthShow.com

www.HolisticCancerFoundation.com

Index

CPSIA information can be obtained
at www.ICGtesting.com
Printed in the USA
BVOW06*0158070817
491017BV00003B/5/P